CRASH COURSE
Neurology

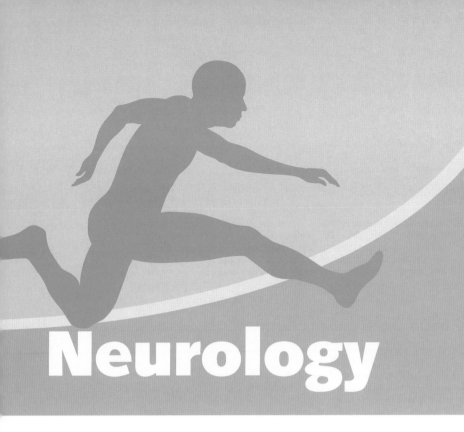

Neurology

Joyce Liporace, MD

Director, Women's Health in Epilepsy Program,
Center for Neuroscience,
Riddle Health Care Center,
Media, Pennsylvania

UK edition authors
Anish Bahra and Katia Cikurel

ELSEVIER
MOSBY

ELSEVIER
MOSBY

1600 John F. Kennedy Blvd.
Suite 1800
Philadelphia, PA 19103-2899

CRASH COURSE: NEUROLOGY
Copyright 2006, Elsevier, Inc.

ISBN-13: 978-1-4160-2962-5
ISBN-10: 1-4160-2962-1

Notice

Knowledge and best practice in this field are constantly changing. As new research and experience broaden our knowledge, changes in practice, treatment and drug therapy may become necessary or appropriate. Readers are advised to check the most current information provided (i) on procedures featured or (ii) by the manufacturer of each product to be administered, to verify the recommended dose or formula, the method and duration of administration, and contraindications. It is the responsibility of the practitioner, relying on their own experience and knowledge of the patient, to make diagnoses, to determine dosages and the best treatment for each individual patient, and to take all appropriate safety precautions. To the fullest extent of the law, neither the Publisher nor the Author assumes any liability for any injury and/or damage to persons or property arising out of or related to any use of the material contained in this book.

The Publisher

Adapted from Crash Course Neurology by Anish Bahra and Katia Cikurel, ISBN: 0-7234-3141-8. Copyright © Harcourt Brace and Company Limited 1999. Copyright © Elsevier Science Limited, 2002. All rights reserved. Published in 1999 by Mosby, an imprint of Elsevier Science Limited.

The rights of Anish Bahra and Katia Cikurel to be identified as the authors of this work have been asserted by them in accordance with the Copyright, Designs and Patents Act, 1988.

Library of Congress Control Number: 2005052281

Acquisitions Editor: Alex Stibbe
Project Development Manager: Stan Ward
Publishing Services Manager: David Saltzberg
Designer: Andy Chapman
Cover Design: Antbits Illustration
Illustration Manager: Mick Ruddy

Printed in China

Last digit is the print number:
9 8 7 6 5 4 3 2 1

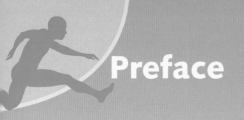

Preface

Neurology is often viewed as extremely complicated and difficult to grasp. Graduating medical students identify the study of neurology as overwhelming. *Crash Course: Neurology* is meant to provide a concise but comprehensive study guide for medical students and residents. Part I of the book presents an analysis and differential diagnosis of common disease symptoms such as dizziness, headache, or weakness. Part II provides a practical guide to taking a history and completing an examination. Part III discusses the presentation and management of the most common neurological diseases affecting the central and peripheral nervous systems.

Medical students should find *Crash Course: Neurology* a handy single source guide during their neurology rotations and also when studying for board examinations. Residents should find that it contains relevant information when caring for patients. I hope that it serves them well.

Joyce Liporace, M.D.

Acknowledgments

I am grateful to the original editors of the UK edition, Anish Bahra and Katia Cikurel. Special thanks to my children, Mike and Matt, and my husband, Tim, for their encouragement and support, and to the Jefferson residents for their inspiration and quest to learn everything about the nervous system.

Contents

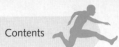

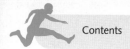

THE PATIENT PRESENTS WITH

Impairment of cognitive (intellectual) function is often a prominent manifestation of cerebral hemisphere disease. The common diffuse or multifocal pathologies in the brain—Alzheimer's or generalized vascular disease, respectively—cause the syndrome of dementia, in which several aspects of cognitive function are impaired. Single localized lesions will predictably cause more focal cognitive deficits, such as aphasia or agnosia. For this reason it is important to be aware of the function of the different lobes and anatomical areas within the cerebral hemispheres. The four lobes—frontal, parietal, temporal, and occipital—are shown in Fig. 1.1. The cerebral cortices have specialized functions. Certain functions are attributes of either the right or left hemisphere; one hemisphere is therefore termed "dominant" and the other "nondominant." The left hemisphere is dominant in over 90% of right-handed people and in about 70% of left-handed people.

Cortical function and clinical manifestations of dysfunction of each lobe are considered below.

The frontal lobe

Function

- The motor cortex. The primary motor cortex is concerned with motor function of the opposite side of the body; the corticospinal and corticobulbar fibers are topographically represented in Fig. 1.2 (termed the homunculus).
- The supplementary motor cortex. This area is concerned with turning of the eyes and head contralaterally.
- Broca's area (dominant hemisphere). Broca's area is the motor center for the production of speech. This is a function of the dominant hemisphere.
- The prefrontal cortex. Personality, emotional expression, initiative, and the ability to plan are governed by the anterior part of the frontal cortex.

- The cortical micturition center. There is normally a cortical inhibition of voiding of the bladder and bowel.

The blood supply to the frontal lobe is from the anterior and middle cerebral arteries, branches of the internal carotid artery.

Lesions of the frontal lobe

Lesions of the frontal lobe give rise to:
- Contralateral mono- or hemiparesis and facial weakness of upper motor neuron type. The pattern of weakness depends on the area of cortex damaged.
- Paralysis of contralateral eye and head turning.
- Broca's expressive aphasia. This consists of nonfluent, hesitant speech with intact comprehension. The patient knows what he or she wants to say but has difficulty finding the correct words, often producing the wrong word. The ability to repeat words is better than spontaneous speech.
- Behavioral change. Features of altered behavior include social disinhibition, loss of initiative and interest, inability to solve problems and loss of abstract thought, and impaired concentration and attention without intellectual or memory decline. This is more common in bilateral lesions. Severe bilateral pathology may result in akinetic mutism, in which the patient is not paralyzed and has the ability to speak but lies still and silent.
- Elicitation of primitive (grasping and sucking) reflexes. These reflexes originate from the parietal cortex and are usually inhibited by the prefrontal cortex.
- Apraxia of gait. This is the inability to walk normally despite preservation of motor and sensory function.
- Incontinence of urine and/or feces. This results from loss of cortical inhibition. There is no desire to micturate. Milder symptoms are frequency and urgency of micturition.

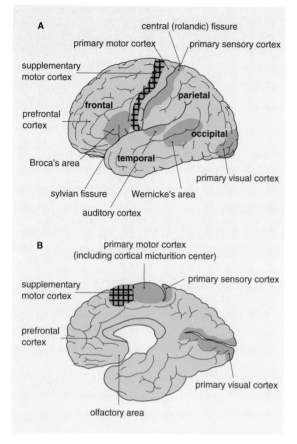

Fig. 1.1 Functional regions of the cerebral cortex. (A) Lateral left hemisphere. (B) Medial right hemisphere.

Focal seizures arising from the frontal cortex give rise to clonic movements of the contralateral lower face, arm, and leg, and conjugate deviation of the head and eyes toward the convulsing side (i.e., away from the side of the lesion).

By virtue of their proximity, lesions of the frontal lobe may be accompanied by disturbance of the olfactory and visual pathways.

The parietal lobe

Function

- The sensory cortex. The parietal cortex receives afferent projections via the thalamus from the somatosensory pathways. The fibers are represented topographically, like the motor pathways.
- Language (dominant hemisphere). Pathways within the arcuate fasciculus connecting Broca's

area (frontal) with Wernicke's area (posterior temporal) pass through the inferior parietal region.
- Use of numbers, as for calculation (dominant hemisphere).
- Integration of somatosensory, visual, and auditory information (mainly nondominant). This allows awareness of the body and its surroundings, appropriate movement of the body, and constructional ability.
- Visual pathways. The upper part of the optic radiation (subserving the lower quadrant of the contralateral visual field) passes deep within the parietal lobe and may be affected in lesions of the deeper white matter.

The blood supply to the parietal lobe is from the middle cerebral artery.

Lesions of the parietal lobe

Lesions of the parietal lobe give rise to:
- Discriminative sensory impairment of the opposite side of the face and limbs. There is impairment of position sense and two-point discrimination, and inability to recognize objects by form and texture (astereognosis) or figures drawn on the hand (agraphesthesia). Pain, temperature, touch, and vibration are intact; however, their localization when applied to the body may be impaired.

Syndromes of the dominant hemisphere

Syndromes of the dominant hemisphere include:
- Gerstmann's syndrome. This consists of confusion of the right and left sides of the body, inability to distinguish the fingers of the hands (finger agnosia), and impairment of calculation (dyscalculia) and writing (dysgraphia). Difficulty with reading (dyslexia) may also occur; this is a function of the dominant parieto-occipital cortex. This lesion occurs with damage to the angular gyrus that spares Wernicke's area.
- Bilateral ideomotor and ideational apraxia. This is the inability to carry out a task on request or by imitation, with normal comprehension and without disturbance of motor or sensory function.

Syndromes of the nondominant hemisphere

Syndromes of the nondominant hemisphere include:

Fig. 1.2 Topographical distribution of the sensorimotor pathways (homunculus).

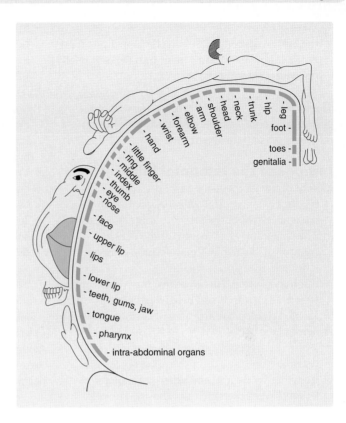

- Constructional apraxia (visuospatial dysfunction). There is difficulty in drawing simple objects (e.g., a house) and with construction (e.g., using building blocks).
- Dressing apraxia. There is difficulty with putting on clothes.
- Contralateral sensory inattention. There is neglect of the opposite side of the body; this may be motor, sensory, or visual (e.g., a hemiplegic patient may ignore the paralyzed side or there may be denial of the hemiplegia). Sensory and visual neglect are discussed in Chapter 14.
- Visual disturbances. If the deeper fibers of the parietal lobe are involved, a contralateral homonymous inferior quadrantanopia (one-fourth of the visual field) and ipsilateral loss of optikokinetic nystagmus may arise. Smooth pursuit eye movements may become "broken."

Focal seizures of the parietal cortex manifest as sensory symptoms of the contralateral side of the body. Descriptions of various sensations may be given (e.g., "pins and needles," tingling), and the symptoms often "march" to adjacent areas of the body.

The temporal lobe

Function

- Wernicke's area (dominant hemisphere). This area is concerned with comprehension of written and spoken language.
- The auditory and vestibular cortex. The primary auditory cortex receives fibers arranged in order of frequency of tone. The auditory pathways from each ear project to both auditory cortices. The dominant temporal lobe is important for the comprehension of spoken words, and the nondominant for the appreciation of sounds and music. Vestibular fibers terminate just posterior to the auditory cortex.
- The limbic lobe. The olfactory and gustatory cortices lie in the medial temporal lobe. The limbic system is important in memory, learning, and emotion.

- Visual pathways. The fibers of the lower part of the optic radiation (subserving the upper quadrant of the contralateral visual field) pass deep through the white matter of the temporal lobe.

The blood supply to the temporal lobe is from the posterior cerebral (medial part of the lobe) and middle cerebral (lateral part) arteries.

Lesions of the temporal lobe

Lesions of the temporal lobe give rise to:

- Cortical deafness. This will only occur with bilateral lesions of the primary auditory cortices. The patient may be unaware of the deficit. Auditory hallucinations may occur in temporal lobe epilepsy.
- Auditory agnosia. This is the inability to recognize sounds (e.g., ringing of a bell, whistling of a kettle, a melody). It occurs in lesions of the nondominant hemisphere.
- Wernicke's receptive aphasia (temporoparietal region). Wernicke's receptive aphasia arises from inferior parietal and superior temporal lesions (Wernicke's area and above). There is impaired comprehension of speech and written language without difficulty with expression. The speech is fluent but words are replaced with partly correct words (word salad), incorrect words related to the words intended (paraphrasia), or newly created meaningless words (neologisms). Thus the speech does not make sense, but the patient has poor insight into the problem. Repetition is poor.

Note that with auditory agnosia and Wernicke's receptive aphasia the function of hearing is normal.

- Vestibular dysfunction. Vestibular dysfunction from a lesion of the vestibular cortex is uncommon, but vertigo may occur as part of the aura of temporal lobe seizures.
- Olfactory and gustatory hallucinations. Olfactory hallucinations and, less commonly, gustatory hallucinations may arise from lesions within the medial temporal lobe, particularly during seizures.
- Learning difficulties. Learning difficulties with auditory information occur in dominant hemisphere lesions; learning difficulties with visual information occur in nondominant hemisphere lesions.

- Memory impairment. This occurs with lesions of the medial temporal lobe involving the hippocampus and parahippocampal gyrus. Bilateral damage results in marked impairment of retention of new information.
- Emotional disturbances. Emotional disturbances from damage to the limbic system may include aggression and rage, apathy, and hypersexuality.
- Visual disturbances. A lesion involving the deeper fibers within the temporal lobe will cause a contralateral superior homonymous quadrantanopia. Complex (or formed) visual hallucinations can occur in temporal lobe seizures.

Temporal lobe seizures may begin with a prodrome of auditory, olfactory, gustatory, or visual hallucinations, a sensation of anxiety or fear, and often a rising epigastric sensation. There may be disturbances of memory, with feelings of familiarity (déjà vu) or unfamiliarity (jamais vu). Behavioral changes may occur; aggression and hypersexuality are reported but are uncommon.

Aphasia

Aphasia is a disorder of spoken and written language; it occurs with damage of the frontal, parietal, or temporal cortices. Broca's expressive and Wernicke's receptive aphasias occur with damage of the dominant hemisphere and have been discussed (see p. 3 and p. 6). The cortical areas subserving these functions are linked by the arcuate fasciculus, which runs in the subcortical white matter. This enables the comprehension of language with subsequent production of speech in response.

- Conduction aphasia occurs with damage to the arcuate fasciculus. The speech is fluent but "jargon" with paraphrasia and neologisms as in Wernicke's aphasia. However, comprehension of language is intact, the patient is aware of the problem, and repetition is markedly impaired.
- Global aphasia occurs with lesions of both Broca's and Wernicke's areas. There is a combination of nonfluent speech and impaired comprehension of language.
- Anomia is an inability to name objects and arises from a lesion of the dominant temporoparietal cortex. It may occur during recovery from the aforementioned aphasias.

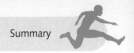

The occipital lobe

Function
The function of the occipital cortex (Fig. 1.3) is the perception of vision and recognition of whatever is visualized. The blood supply is from the posterior cerebral artery, but the occipital poles have additional supply from a branch of the middle cerebral artery.

Lesions of the occipital lobe
Lesions of the occipital lobe give rise to:
- Contralateral homonymous hemianopic field defect. If this arises from a lesion of the posterior cerebral artery, there will be sparing of the macular area. A lesion of the occipital pole will affect the macular fibers only and result in a contralateral homonymous hemianopic macular field defect.
- Cortical blindness. Bilateral occipital lesions render the patient blind, with retention of the pupillary reflexes. The patient may deny the blindness (Anton's syndrome).
- Visual agnosia. Lesions of the visual association cortices cause impairment of recognition of faces and objects.
- Visual illusions. Objects may appear larger (macropsia) or smaller (micropsia); there may be disturbances of shape, color, and number. This is more common with lesions of the nondominant hemisphere.

Visual hallucinations in seizures of the primary visual cortex are unformed (flashes of light and geometric shapes); those due to seizure activity from the visual association cortex or its connections with the temporal cortex are formed (objects, people).

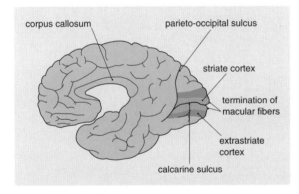

Fig. 1.3 The occipital lobe. The striate (primary visual) and extrastriate (visual association) cortices are shown, and termination of the macular fibers at the poles.

Summary

Focal damage to the cerebral hemispheres usually results from vascular events (infarction or hemorrhage), tumors, trauma, or localized inflammatory lesions (e.g., abscess, tuberculoma). Generalized or multifocal cerebral dysfunction results most often from degenerative dementias (Alzheimer's disease, Pick's disease), multiple infarcts, demyelination, or diffuse infections (encephalitis, meningitis).

Fig. 1.4. summarizes the symptoms that may arise from focal lesions of the cerebral hemisphere.

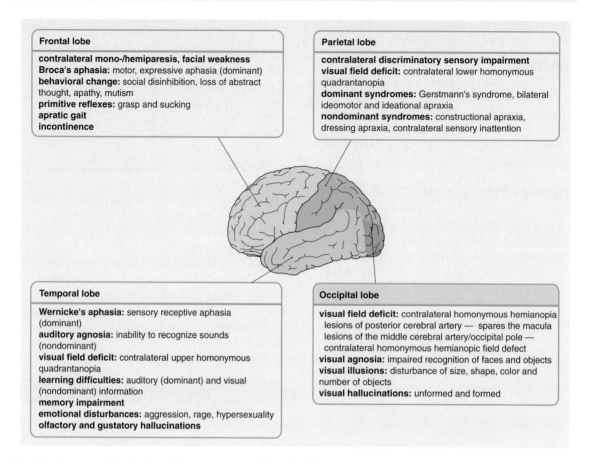

Frontal lobe

contralateral mono-/hemiparesis, facial weakness
Broca's aphasia: motor, expressive aphasia (dominant)
behavioral change: social disinhibition, loss of abstract thought, apathy, mutism
primitive reflexes: grasp and sucking
apratic gait
incontinence

Parietal lobe

contralateral discriminatory sensory impairment
visual field deficit: contralateral lower homonymous quadrantanopia
dominant syndromes: Gerstmann's syndrome, bilateral ideomotor and ideational apraxia
nondominant syndromes: constructional apraxia, dressing apraxia, contralateral sensory inattention

Temporal lobe

Wernicke's aphasia: sensory receptive aphasia (dominant)
auditory agnosia: inability to recognize sounds (nondominant)
visual field deficit: contralateral upper homonymous quadrantanopia
learning difficulties: auditory (dominant) and visual (nondominant) information
memory impairment
emotional disturbances: aggression, rage, hypersexuality
olfactory and gustatory hallucinations

Occipital lobe

visual field deficit: contralateral homonymous hemianopia lesions of posterior cerebral artery — spares the macula lesions of the middle cerebral artery/occipital pole — contralateral homonymous hemianopic field defect
visual agnosia: impaired recognition of faces and objects
visual illusions: disturbance of size, shape, color and number of objects
visual hallucinations: unformed and formed

Fig. 1.4 Summary of localization of symptoms arising from focal lesions of the cerebral hemispheres.

2. Disturbances of Consciousness

Transient loss of consciousness

Transient loss or disturbance of consciousness is a very common presenting problem. Usually the patient has no symptoms or physical signs when seen, and subsequent investigations are often normal. The diagnosis is therefore critically dependent on a careful history taken from the patient and from any available witness. Recurrent loss of consciousness is usually due to epilepsy, vasovagal syncope, or cardiac arrhythmia.

Syncope

The conscious state is maintained by the cerebral cortex and brainstem reticular formation. Syncope is the transient loss of consciousness and posture that results from a global reduction in blood flow to the brain.

Vasovagal syncope

In vasovagal syncope, the sudden drop in blood pressure results from "peripheral" vasodilatation. There is a subsequent reduction in cardiac output, which is followed by vagal stimulation and thus bradycardia. Typical precipitating situations are strong emotion, sudden intense pain, and prolonged standing in hot, crowded areas.

Notably, the patient is usually upright at the onset of syncope. Prodromal symptoms include feeling light-headed, gradual dimming of vision, ringing in the ears, salivation, sweating, nausea, and sometimes vomiting. These symptoms may last from several seconds to a few minutes. The attack can be aborted if the patient assumes the supine position, otherwise consciousness is subsequently lost. The patient is pale and clammy, the pulse almost imperceptible, and the systolic blood pressure drops to about 60 mmHg. If this state persists for sufficient time to cause cerebral hypoxia, the eyes may roll upward and there may be brief convulsive movements, which can be mistaken for a seizure. However, sphincter control is almost invariably maintained and a typical postictal picture is not seen, although there may be prolonged fatigue afterward.

Micturition and cough syncope

Micturition syncope occurs in men who get up during the night to pass urine. It results from a combination of vasodilatation (which occurs with emptying of the bladder), a degree of postural hypotension on standing, and bradycardia. The loss of consciousness is sudden, with an equally rapid recovery.

Sustained coughing can elevate the intrathoracic pressure sufficiently to impair the venous return to the heart. Increase of the cerebrospinal fluid pressure, reduction of PCO_2, and resultant vasoconstriction may also be contributory. The mechanism behind the Valsalva maneuver (exhalation against a closed glottis) is similar and is that seen in syncope following breath-holding attacks in children and strenuous activity (e.g., heavy lifting or laughing).

Postural hypotension

In a number of clinical conditions, the upright posture is accompanied by an uncompensated fall in blood pressure and therefore also cerebral blood flow. Postural hypotension may occur:

- In normal individuals.
- After a debilitating illness with recumbency.
- In patients with large varicose veins in which there is significant venous pooling.
- In autonomic neuropathy (e.g., diabetes, Guillain Barré syndrome, amyloidosis).
- In hypovolemia (e.g., loss of blood, diuretic therapy, Addison's disease).
- With drugs (e.g., antihypertensives).

Syncope of cardiac origin

Syncope of cardiac origin is usually abrupt and without prodrome. The upright position is not a prerequisite. Loss of consciousness is brief and classically accompanied by marked pallor with a

9

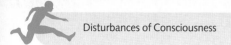

rapid return of color as cardiac output is restored. (Pallor is prolonged after vasovagal syncope.) Brief tonic or clonic movements may occur, but recovery is usually rapid. The examination and further investigation with 24-hour electrocardiogram (ECG) monitoring and an echocardiogram will further support the history, suggesting a cardiac cause. These include:

- Cardiac arrhythmias (usually profound bradycardia).
- Left ventricular outflow obstruction—aortic stenosis, hypertrophic obstructive cardiomyopathy.
- Right ventricular outflow obstruction—pulmonary stenosis, pulmonary hypertension, pulmonary embolism.
- Ventricular failure.

Seizures

The most common diagnostic problem is distinguishing a syncopal attack from an epileptic seizure. Certain features of the clinical picture aid the differentiation between the two:

- A seizure can occur in any position. Syncopal attacks tend to occur in the upright position, although this is less so with those of cardiac origin, particularly Stokes–Adams attacks (syncope due to transient complete heart block).
- The onset of a seizure is more sudden. There may be preceding aura symptoms but these usually last only seconds, shorter than the characteristic prodrome of syncope. The notable exception is the abrupt onset of a Stokes–Adams attack.
- Urinary incontinence often accompanies a seizure but is rare with syncope. Fecal incontinence can occur with a seizure but not with a syncopal attack.
- During a seizure, patients may bite their tongue.
- Following recovery from a seizure, the patient may be confused, drowsy, and with headache. The patient recovers consciousness and orientation more rapidly from a syncopal attack, but there may be prolonged fatigue afterward.
- Injury is more common consequent to a seizure.

The different types of seizure are dealt with in more detail in Chapter 21.

If a seizure is suspected, electroencephalography (EEG) may give information about the presence of abnormal epileptiform activity, but it is not a diagnostic test. The EEG is often normal in patients

with seizures. The diagnosis is made primarily from the history and an eye-witness account of the event. Imaging studies with magnetic resonance (MR) or computed tomography (CT) are complementary.

- Diagnosis of epilepsy is *clinical*, based on the history or on direct observation of attacks.
- An EEG can only lend support to the clinical diagnosis or help to classify seizure types. Often it is normal or unremarkable.

Further differential diagnoses

In patients presenting with episodes of transient loss of consciousness, the first step is to establish whether the attacks may have been syncopal or a seizure. The history is most important. Thereafter, further differential diagnoses may be considered (Fig. 2.1):

- Vertebrobasilar ischemia.
- Carotid sinus disease.
- Hyperventilation.
- Narcolepsy and cataplexy.
- Hypoglycemia.
- Vertebrobasilar migraine.
- Psychogenic seizures.

Cerebrovascular disease

The brainstem reticular formation is supplied by the vertebrobasilar arterial tree. Compromise of this blood supply may result in loss of consciousness as part of a brainstem transient ischemic attack. Associated symptoms of brainstem origin, such as vertigo and diplopia, are necessary for the diagnosis (e.g., subclavian steal syndrome, Takayasu's disease [aortic arch syndrome], thromboembolic predisposition). Similar symptoms may occur in vertebrobasilar migraine.

Carotid sinus disease

The carotid sinus responds to stretch (via a branch of the glossopharyngeal nerve and thence the medulla) by producing a reflex bradycardia or a reduction in arterial pressure without the bradycardia. A syncopal attack may ensue in patients with carotid sinus hypersensitivity. Characteristically, this occurs if the patient turns his or her head toward one side or if the carotid sinuses are massaged.

Differential diagnosis of transient loss of consciousness

Seizure	Syncope	
can occur in any position and time of day preceding aura symptoms sudden onset urinary or fecal incontinence tongue biting postictal confusion, drowsiness, and headache	upright position usually prodrome—light headed, nausea, ringing in ears, dimming of vision, pallor, sweating hypotension and thready pulse relatively rapid recovery	
	Situational emotion or pain micturition coughing postural	*Cardiac* left or right ventricular outflow obstruction arrhythmia "pump" failure
Further differential diagnoses	**Clinical features**	
vertebrobasilar ischemia	additional brainstem symptoms, e.g., verligo, diplopia cerebrovascular risk factors, e.g., hypertension, diabetes, ischemic heart disease check peripheral upper limb pulses	
carotid sinus disease	syncope on turning head or on neck massage postural hypotension confirmed on tilt-table testing	
hyperventilation	anxiety or situational, e.g., crowded rooms perioral and/or digital tingling, carpopedal spasm, chest pain high respiratory rate, low PCO_2, metabolic alkalosis	
narcolepsy/cataplexy	inappropriate desire to sleep falls with emotional situations, e.g., laughing family history and presence of HLA-DR2	
hypoglycemia	diabetic on treatment or relative of such a patient hepatic failure hypopituitarism, Addison's disease insulinoma glycogen storage disease excess alcohol ideal diagnosis is the documentation of a low blood glucose whilst symptomatic	
miscellaneous vertebrobasilar migraine psychogenic seizure	look for a history of headache and other brainstem symptoms a diagnosis of exclusion	

Fig. 2.1 Differential diagnosis of transient loss of consciousness. If a patient presents with episodes of transient loss of consciousness, the first step is to establish whether the attacks are syncopal or due to a seizure. The history is most important. Thereafter further differential diagnoses may be concluded as shown here.

Hyperventilation

Overbreathing results in a reduction of PCO_2, cerebral vasoconstriction, a metabolic alkalosis, and a reduction in ionized calcium. Characteristic features are:

- Breathlessness and air hunger with rapid respiration.
- Light-headedness.
- Perioral and digital paresthesia.
- Carpopedal spasm.
- Variable submammary or axillary chest pain.
- Anxiety and fatigue.

The attacks may occur in particular situations due to phobic anxiety, commonly in crowds or sometimes after physical exertion.

Narcolepsy and cataplexy

Narcolepsy is a recurrent irresistible desire to sleep. It occurs in inappropriate situations. The patient is easily roused and wakes from sleep refreshed (unlike patients with obstructive sleep apnea). It is associated with HLA-DR2.

Cataplexy is a related disorder whereby the patient has a tendency to collapse and fall with transient loss of muscle tone but fully preserved consciousness. Attacks are provoked by strong emotion such as laughter, surprise, or anger. Recovery is immediate.

Hypoglycemia

Hypoglycemia is accompanied by a surge in catecholamine secretion. Thus the patient begins to feel hunger; there is a tremor, sweating, palpitations, confusion, and ultimately loss of consciousness. Seizures often occur as a secondary phenomenon.

Coma

Coma is a state of impaired consciousness in which the patient is not roused by external stimuli. Inattention, confusion, stupor, and coma are terms describing progressive states of impaired consciousness. However, they are not clearly defined and therefore inter-observer interpretation is highly variable. The Glasgow Coma Scale (Fig. 2.2) provides a more objective and reproducible method by which conscious level can be assessed and documented; it is based on eye opening and verbal and motor responses. A patient with a normal

Glasgow Coma Scale
Eye opening
1　None
2　In response to pain
3　In response to speech
4　Spontaneous
Verbal responses
1　None
2　Incomprehensible sounds
3　Inappropriate words
4　Disorientated speech
5　Orientated speech
Motor responses
1　None
2　Extensor response to pain
3　Flexor response to pain
4　Withdrawal to pain
5　Localization of painful stimulus
6　Obeys commands

Fig. 2.2 The Glasgow Coma Scale.

conscious state will score a total of 15. Note that the lowest possible score is 3.

Differential diagnosis

Certain conditions may resemble coma but should be distinguished from it.

Akinetic mutism

A patient with akinetic mutism is able to comprehend what is occurring around him or her and appears alert, but is silent and does not move spontaneously or respond to external stimuli. This arises from bilateral frontal lobe damage; the corticoreticular pathways are interrupted but the motor and sensory pathways are spared.

Locked-in syndrome

In locked-in syndrome, a lesion of the ventral pons interrupts the corticobulbar and corticospinal pathways, with sparing of the reticular pathways. The patient is therefore alert but unable to respond with speech or facial or limb movements. The pathways for eye movement are spared, so the patient can respond with vertical eye movements and blinking.

Persistent vegetative state

Persistent vegetative state describes a state in which after severe cerebral injury, patients recover partially

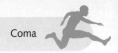

from a comatose state and alternate between a state of wakefulness and nonwakefulness. However, there is no purposeful behavior and no demonstrable cognitive function.

Catatonia

A catatonic patient is silent and there is no volitional motor or emotional response to external stimuli. The patient may resist an examiner's attempt to move, for example, a limb, and if the limb is moved, the patient may keep it fixed in this position for some time. This may be seen in catatonic schizophrenic states.

Nonconvulsive status epilepticus

Nonconvulsive status epilepticus should be suspected in patients who do not regain consiousness after convulsive status epilepticus. An EEG will confirm subclinical epileptic activity. It may also be seen in epileptic patients with a change in awareness or personality.

Causes of loss or disturbance of consciousness may be intracranial or extracranial (Figs 2.3 and 2.4).

Clinical approach to the comatose patient

The first step is to ascertain whether there is:
- Airway—establish an airway.
- Breathing—ensure that the patient is adequately ventilated with oxygen.
- Circulation—ensure there is cardiac output; otherwise begin external cardiac massage.

If there is circulatory failure, this must be corrected and the potential cause pursued. Once a stable cardiorespiratory status has been established, a history should be taken from a relative, friend, or witness, and a clinical examination and initial investigations must be performed to ascertain the cause of coma.

Examination of the comatose patient

Examine the patient for:
- Signs of head injury.
- Neck stiffness (if no evidence of cervical spine injury).
- Respiratory pattern.
- Pupil responses.
- Ocular movements.
- Fundoscopic abnormalities.
- Limb posture and movement.
- Reflexes and plantar responses.

Respiratory pattern

- Cheyne–Stokes respiration—alternate hyper- and hypoventilation; seen in metabolic and iatrogenic disturbances, and bilateral deep hemisphere lesions (thalamus or internal capsule).
- Central neurogenic hyperventilation—metabolic disturbances, e.g., diabetic and salicylate acidosis, and lesions of the reticular formation.
- Ataxic respiration—irregular respiratory pattern seen in lesions of the medulla.
- Apneustic respiration—pauses of 2–3 seconds occur after inspiration; seen in pontine lesions.

Pupil responses

- Pinpoint—pontine lesion, opiates.
- Bilateral fixed mid-position—midbrain lesion.
- Unilateral or bilateral fixed and dilated—supratentorial mass with uncal herniation.
- Enlarged, slowly reactive pupils—metabolic or toxic.

Ocular movements

- Oculocephalic reflex—in patients with an intact brainstem, on rotating the head to the left and right, the eyes will move conjugately, opposite to the movement of the head.
- Oculovestibular reflex—pouring cold water into the ear causes deviation of the eyes toward the side irrigated, followed by corrective nystagmus in the opposite direction.
- Lesions of the midbrain or pons may result in dysconjugate movements of the eyes.

Fundoscopic abnormalities

Look for papilledema and subhyaloid hemorrhage.

Limb posture and movement

- Decerebrate posturing—neck extension with extension, abduction, and/or pronation of arms, extension of legs and plantarflexed feet (dEcerebrate = arm Extension).
- Decorticate posturing—flexion and/or adduction of arms, extension of legs.

Investigations in the comatose patient

Immediate investigations include:
- Temperature.
- Blood glucose.
- Electrolytes, calcium, and urea and creatinine.
- Complete blood count and coagulation screen.
- Arterial blood gases.

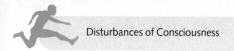

Intracranial causes of loss or disturbance of consciousness		
Intracranial cause	**Clinical features**	**Investigations**
epilepsy	convulsive movements incontinence tongue biting	EEG
trauma extradural hemorrhage	evidence of head injury—laceration, bruising, blood or CSF from nose or ear	fracture on skull x-ray CT or MRI of head
subdural hemorrhage	past history of head injury several weeks previously; the elderly and alcoholics are prone to falls	CT or MRI of head
Vascular subarachnoid hemorrhage	history of explosive-onset headache collapse subhyaloid hemorrhage pyrexia neck stiffness, +ve Kernig's sign focal neurological signs if there is intracerebral extension of the blood	CT of head—should be performed within 48 hours to avoid false negative results lumbar puncture (LP)—if CT is normal, an LP should be done between 12 hours and 1 week after the initial event—xanthochromic CSF
intracerebral hemorrhage	collapse	CT or MRI of head
hypertensive encephalopathy	hypertension, retinopathy, seizures	
vertebrobasilar thromboembolism	history of TIAs or stroke, valvular or ischemic heart disease, predisposition to thromboembolism	
Infective meningitis	headache pyrexia neck stiffness, +ve Kernig's sign maculopapular body rash	if there is no evidence of raised intracranial pressure, an LP should be done; otherwise CT should be performed first
encephalitis		CT or MRI—focal or diffuse cerebral edema EEG LP
cerebral abscess	subacute onset headache usually focal symptoms and signs often seizures source of infection elsewhere—ears, sinuses, lungs, valvular heart disease	CT or MRI of head blood cultures microbiology from potential source of infection

Fig. 2.3 Intracranial causes of loss or disturbance of consciousness.

Extracranial causes of loss or disturbance of consciousness		
Extracranial cause	**Clinical features**	**Investigations**
Circulatory collapse cardiac, e.g. arrhythmia, myocardial infarction	hypotension, tachycardia, rhythm disturbance, cardiac failure	ECG, cardiac enzymes, echocardiogram
septicemic shock	rigors, pyrexia, vomiting, peripheral vasodilatation	cultures—blood, sputum, urine, throat, stool
hypovolemia, e.g. blood loss profuse diarrhea	melena, hematemesis, abdominal pain (ruptured aortic aneurysm)	
hypotensive drugs		
Metabolic hypo- or hypernatremia	**subacute onset** muscle twitches, dehydration	
hypo- or hyperkalemia	cardiac muscle excitability, ileus, diabetes insipidus	
hypo- or hypercalcemia	carpopedal spasm polyuria and/or polydipsia, abdominal pain, vomiting	biochemical confirmation
hypo- or hyperglycemia	hemiplegia [reversible], seizures dehydration, hyperventilation, ketotic smell	
hypo- or hyperthermia	bradycardia, hypotension, hypoventilation, rigidity, cardiac arrest	rectal temperature
uremia	sallow skin, uremic smell, pale conjunctiva, hypertension	raised creatinine, acidosis, anemia
hepatic failure	jaundice, signs of portal hypertension, GI bleed, sedative drugs, sepsis	abnormal LFIs, raised ammonia, electrolyte imbalance
hypoxia	following respiratory failure, cardiorespiratory arrest; brain damage occurs after 4 minutes of anoxia	
hypercapnia	pink puffer, bounding pulse, papilledema, asterixis	elevated PCO_2
Endocrine adrenal crisis	hypotension, abdominal pain, buccal and flexure pigmentation	low Na^+, Ca^{2+}, glucose raised K^+, ACTH stimulation test
hypopituitarism	pallor, hypogonadism, bitemporal hemianopia	low pituitary and target hormones, CT/MRI of head
myxedema	dry and coarse facies, hypotension, bradycardia, hypothermia	clinical diagnosis confirmed by thyroid function tests; pituitary failure
hypo- or hyperparathyroidism	as for hypo- and hyperthyroidism	$\downarrow/\uparrow Ca^{2+}$, $\downarrow/\uparrow$ parathyroid hormone
Toxins alcohol	ethanolic smell Wernicke's encephalopathy	raised blood alcohol level low thiamine
carbon monoxide	red skin color	elevated carboxyhemoglobin
Drugs opiates	slow respiratory rate, pin-point pupils	reversible with naloxone +ve blood and urine toxicology
sedatives	barbiturates—hypotension and hypothermia	+ve toxicology
tricyclic antidepressants	dilated pupils with sluggish responses, hypothermia	
Psychiatric catatonia	as described above (p. 13)	
psychogenic	eyelids resist opening; normal reflexes and plantar responses; corneal reflex cannot be suppressed; normal caloric response	

Fig. 2.4 Extracranial causes of loss or disturbance of consciousness.

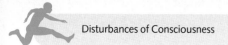
- Blood culture and toxicology.
- ECG and chest x-ray.

Neurologic investigations in selected cases include:
- Brain imaging (CT or MR imaging).

- Cerebrospinal fluid examination.
- EEG.

Examination of brainstem reflexes used in the diagnosis of brain death are listed in Fig. 2.5.

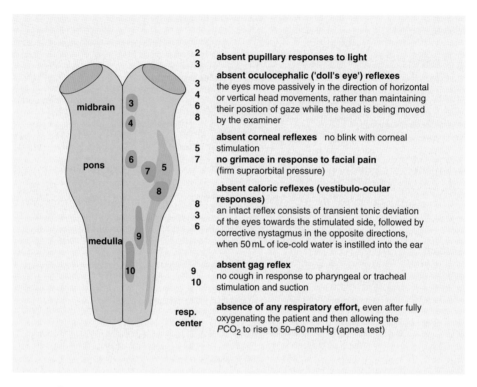

Fig. 2.5 Brainstem reflexes used in the diagnosis of brain death. Note that examination findings in the limbs are not relevant. The tendon reflexes may be intact, since these occur at spinal levels. There may also be limb posturing to painful stimuli in some cases. The examination should be repeated within 24 hours by a second experienced clinician to confirm that irreversible brain death has occurred. Some centers require confirmatory tests, such as EEG, blood flow, or brainstem auditory evoked potentials (BAEPs), especially in cases of organ donation.

3. Headache

Most patients with headaches have tension-type or migraine headache; the diagnosis in such cases is made entirely from the history because there are no physical signs. However, headache may also be secondary to other disorders affecting the head and neck, and it is sometimes the predominant symptom of serious intracranial disease—usually vascular, infective, or neoplastic.

Pain may be referred from the ears, eyes, nasal passages, teeth, sinuses, facial bones, or cervical spine. It is conveyed predominantly by the trigeminal nerve (fifth cranial nerve), and also by the seventh, ninth, and tenth cranial nerves, and the upper three cervical roots. Generally, structures of the anterior and middle cranial fossa refer pain to the anterior two-thirds of the head via the branches of the trigeminal nerve; structures of the posterior fossa refer pain to the back of the head and neck via the upper cervical roots (Fig. 3.1).

Differential diagnosis

The approach to assessing a patient with headache should be based on the temporal pattern of symptoms, especially the mode of onset and subsequent course. This may be:
- Recurrent and episodic.
- Chronic and daily.
- Subacute onset.
- Acute onset.

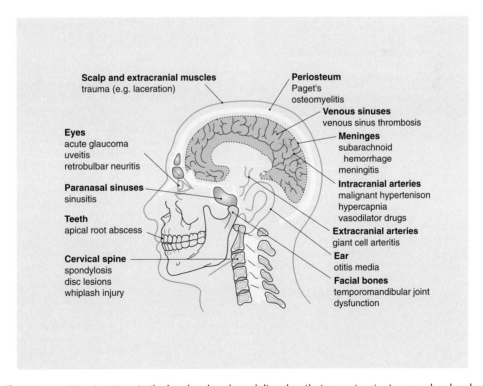

Scalp and extracranial muscles
trauma (e.g. laceration)

Periosteum
Paget's
osteomyelitis

Venous sinuses
venous sinus thrombosis

Eyes
acute glaucoma
uveitis
retrobulbar neuritis

Meninges
subarachnoid
hemorrhage
meningitis

Intracranial arteries
malignant hypertenison
hypercapnia
vasodilator drugs

Paranasal sinuses
sinusitis

Teeth
apical root abscess

Extracranial arteries
giant cell arteritis

Ear
otitis media

Cervical spine
spondylosis
disc lesions
whiplash injury

Facial bones
temporomandibular joint
dysfunction

Fig. 3.1 The pain-sensitive structures in the head and neck, and disorders that may give rise to secondary headache.

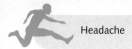

Recurrent episodic headache
Recurrent episodic headache is usually benign and is very rarely due to structural or progressive pathology. Common causes and their clinical features are listed in Fig. 3.2.

Chronic daily headache
Chronic daily headache is most often diffuse tension-type headache and, again, is rarely due to serious intracranial disease (Fig. 3.3).

Subacute-onset headache
The category of subacute-onset headache includes most of the serious causes of headache. Worrying features include a progressive course, persisting focal symptoms or signs, deterioration of conscious level, seizures, or associated fever (Fig. 3.4).

Acute-onset headache
Instantaneous onset should always raise the suspicion of intracranial hemorrhage, although there are other causes, as listed in Fig. 3.5.

History

A good history is essential to the diagnosis of the type of headache. Determine:
- Mode of onset—acute, subacute, chronic, or recurrent and episodic.

Recurrent episodic headache	
Cause	Clinical features
migraine	unilateral throbbing headache exacerbated by movement accompanied by nausea, vomiting, photo-, phono- and osmophobia +/− aura symptoms
cluster headache	severe unilateral retro-orbital +/− temporal pain; ipsilateral conjunctival injection, lacrimation, partial Horner's syndrome, nasal blockage, rhinorrhea; attacks last 15–180 minutes and occur several times a day for about 2–3 months at a time
trigeminal neuralgia	jabs of severe unilateral pain in the 2nd and 3rd distribution of the trigeminal nerve; triggered by actions such as chewing, brushing teeth, talking, cold wind
benign exertional/cough headache	headaches precipitated by exertion, coughing, straining and sexual activity; may be benign, but this diagnosis is one of exclusion
intermittent hydrocephalus	intermittent severe headaches accompanied by drop attacks, weakness of the legs and unsteady gait, e.g., intermittent obstruction of the third ventricle by a colloid cyst
paroxysmal hypertension	this may occur in patients with a pheochromocytoma

Fig. 3.2 Differential diagnosis of recurrent episodic headache.

Chronic daily headache	
Cause	Clinical features
transformed migraine +/− analgesic overuse	daily, mild, bilateral, usually featureless headache with superimposed episodes of characteristic migraine headaches
tension-type headache +/− analgesic overuse	bilateral featureless headache; usually episodic
postherpetic neuralgia	after an attack of herpes zoster there may be continuous burning pain with superimposed occasional stabs in the distribution of the affected nerve(s)
posttraumatic headache	posttraumatic headache syndromes include: post-concussion headache; episodic headaches which may be migrainous; generalized featureless daily headache; tenderness or pain located to the site of the injury; occipital and/or neck pain from upper cervical spine injury
atypical facial pain	constant aching pain in the lower part of the face more commonly occurs in women; it may follow a minor facial injury or dental procedure

Fig. 3.3 Differential diagnosis of chronic daily headache.

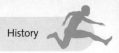

Subacute-onset headache	
Cause	Clinical features
subdural hematoma	history of head injury (elderly and alcoholics in particular), fluctuating level of consciousness, confusion, focal neurological signs (usually a hemiparesis)
intracranial tumor	headache exacerbated by coughing, sneezing, or straining may occur with obstruction of the CSF pathways focal neurological signs, seizures
intracranial abscess	direct extension from local disease (e.g., frontal sinusitis) or metastatic spread (e.g., lung abscess) fever, systemically unwell, focal neurological signs the above can be diagnosed on CT or MRI
chronic meningitis	tuberculosis (note ethnic origin and HIV status), cryptococcal (HIV), malignant, syphilitic, sarcoid
giant-cell arteritis	patients usually over 50 years of age; female preponderance visual disturbance–ischemic papillopathy associated polymyalgia rheumatica elevated ESR tender thickened superficial temporal artery; giant-cell arteritis on biopsy urgent steroid therapy often prior to biopsy
benign intracranial hypertension	young, overweight females papilledema, raised CSF pressure CT or MRI usually normal, although the lateral ventricles often appear small

Fig. 3.4 Differential diagnosis of subacute-onset headache.

- Subsequent course—episodic, progressive, or chronic and persistent.
- Site—unilateral or bilateral; frontal, temporal, or occipital; radiation to neck, arm, or shoulder.
- Character of pain—constant, throbbing, stabbing, or dull/pressure-like.
- Frequency and duration.
- Accompanying features—additional neurological symptoms, neck stiffness, autonomic symptoms.

Acute-onset headache	
Cause	Clinical features
subarachnoid hemorrhage	explosive-onset "thunderclap headache" neck stiffness, photophobia, +ve Kernig's sign +/– focal neurological signs if there has been intracerebral extension of blood CT head scan—subarachnoid blood (within 48 hours) CSF—xanthochromia (12 hours to 1 week)
cerebral hemorrhage	note history of hypertension, anticoagulation focal neurological signs depending on site of bleed CT head scan—intracerebral blood
meningitis/encephalitis	+/– history of recent respiratory tract infection fever, neck stiffness, +ve Kernig's sign inflammatory CSF
acute hydrocephalus	nausea, vomiting, diplopia (6th nerve palsy—false localizing sign) +/– papilledema, ataxia of gait diagnosis confirmed on CT head scan
hypertensive crisis	very high blood pressure there may be papilledema there may be other features of pheochromocytoma
acute glaucoma	pain typically frontal, orbital or ocular, accompanied by persisting visual impairment, fixed oval pupil and conjunctival injection this is an ophthalmological emergency
first episode of migraine/cluster headache	migraine can present with an explosive "thunderclap" onset; the diagnosis of a migrainous etiology is then one of exclusion, unless recurrent stereotyped episodes have occurred over several years.

Fig. 3.5 Differential diagnosis of acute-onset headache.

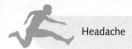
- Exacerbating factors—movement, light, noise, smell (e.g., migraine); coughing, sneezing, bending (e.g., raised intracranial pressure).
- Precipitating factors—alcohol (cluster headache and migraine), menstruation (migraine), stress (most headaches are worse with stress), postural change (high or low intracranial pressure), head injury (subdural hemorrhage or posttraumatic headache).
- Particular time of onset—mornings (migraine, raised intracranial pressure), awoken at night (cluster headache).
- Past history of headache.
- Family history—migraine, hypertension, intracranial hemorrhage.
- General health—systemic ill-health, existing medical conditions.
- Drug history—analgesic abuse, recreational drugs.

Examination

When examining a patient with headache, look for:
- Focal neurologic signs.
- Signs of local disease of the ears, eyes, or sinuses; restriction of neck movements and pain; temporomandibular dysfunction; thickening of the superficial temporal arteries.
- Signs of systemic disease.
- Abnormal blood pressure.

Remember, the clinical examination is often entirely normal.

Summary

Headache may be:
- Primary (e.g., migraine, tension-type headache, cluster headache).

- Secondary (e.g., subarachnoid hemorrhage, meningitis, raised intracranial pressure).

First, the temporal pattern of symptoms should be established, i.e., the mode of onset and subsequent course—recurrent and episodic, chronic, subacute, or acute. A list of differential diagnoses of the possible causes should come to mind based on the established temporal pattern of symptoms. The history and examination should further narrow the differential diagnoses and indicate which patients may have a secondary headache.

Features that should alert the clinician to the presence of a secondary headache and prompt further investigation are:
- Recent onset/short history (particularly in middle age with no previous history of headache).
- Recent change in established pattern or character of headache.
- Increasing severity with resistance to appropriate and adequately tried treatment.
- Associated features—neurologic signs, seizures, personality change, fever, systemic ill-health.

Alteration of the sense of smell is not a common presenting symptom, and impairment of olfaction as a physical sign is not often important in making a neurologic diagnosis. Consequently, smell is not always tested during a routine clinical examination. However, anosmia is a significant problem after some head injuries, and, in rare cases, it can be the only physical sign of a serious structural lesion involving the frontal lobes.

Afferent impulses conveying information about various odors are conveyed by the receptor cells of the nasal mucosa. These are bipolar neurons that have peripheral and central processes. The peripheral processes contain many cilia, which carry the olfactory receptors. The unmyelinated central processes pass into the cranial cavity through the cribiform plate of the ethmoid bone to synapse in the olfactory bulb; these fibers constitute the first (olfactory) nerve. Axons from the olfactory bulb form the olfactory tract. This tract runs in the olfactory groove of the cribiform plate beneath the frontal lobes and above the optic nerve and chiasm. The fibers synapse within the anterior perforated substance and ultimately terminate in the primary olfactory cortex (in the anterior aspect of the hippocampal gyrus and uncus of the temporal lobe) and nuclei of the amygdaloid complex (Fig. 4.1).

The anosmia or hyposmia may be temporary or permanent. Note that if the impairment of olfaction is unilateral, it will not be noticed by the patient. Olfaction tends to deteriorate with age.

The following causes should be considered:
- Upper respiratory tract infection—chronic rhinitis, sinusitis (allergic, vasomotor, or infective).
- Heavy smoking.
- Viral infections—e.g., influenza, herpes simplex (may cause permanent destruction of the receptor cells).
- Drugs—e.g., antibiotics, antihistamines.
- Local trauma to the olfactory epithelium.
- Head injury—fibers from the receptor cells are damaged during their passage through the cribriform plate, particularly if there is an associated fracture. If the dura is torn, there may be cerebrospinal fluid rhinorrhea; this can be differentiated from mucous secretion by its higher glucose concentration.
- Tumors—meningioma of the olfactory groove may extend posteriorly to involve the optic nerve; frontal lobe and pituitary tumors.
- Aneurysm of the anterior cerebral or anterior communicating artery.
- Raised intracranial pressure—olfaction may be impaired without evidence of damage to the olfactory structures.

Differential diagnosis

Anosmia and hyposmia

Anosmia is loss of the sense of smell. Hyposmia is impairment of the sense of smell. Anosmia or hyposmia may be due to:
- Inability of odors to reach the olfactory receptors (hypertrophy or hyperemia of the nasal mucosa).
- Destruction of the receptor cells.
- A central lesion.

Ageusia and hypogeusia

Ageusia is the perception of loss of taste. Hypogeusia is the perception of an impaired sense of taste.

Many patients with bilateral anosmia complain of loss or impairment of taste. This is because much of our appreciation of food and drink is by olfaction rather than by elemental taste. Taste itself is normal if tested formally in anosmic subjects.

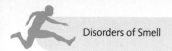

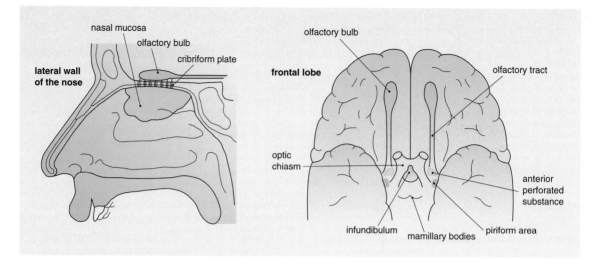

Fig. 4.1 The anatomic relations of the olfactory nerve.

Hyperosmia

Hyperosmia is an abnormally increased sensitivity to odors and may be seen in the following conditions:

- Neurotic individuals may complain of hypersensitivity to various odors.
- Migraine attacks with and without aura may be accompanied by hypersensitivity to light, sound, and smell (osmophobia).

Olfactory hallucinations

- Complex partial seizures of temporal lobe origin can give rise to brief olfactory hallucinations, which are part of the aura.
- Olfactory hallucinations may occur following alcohol withdrawal.
- Olfactory hallucinations and delusions of unpleasant nature are often due to a psychotic illness (e.g., depression or schizophrenia).
- Hallucinations and delusions may also occur in patients with dementia.

A persistent unpleasant smell may occur from local disease of the nasopharynx such as purulent sinusitis.

Disorders of smell:

- Anosmia/hyposmia is the loss/impairment of smell. This is noticed by the patient if the impairment is bilateral but not if unilateral.
- Ageusia/hypogeusia is an apparent alteration in taste perception in individuals with bilateral anosmia.
- Hyperosmia is a hypersensitivity to odors.
- Olfactory hallucinations may occur with temporal lobe seizures, following alcohol withdrawal, or as a manifestation of psychosis or in patients with dementia.

Examination

A characteristic-smelling object (e.g., peppermint, clove oil) is held under each nostril in turn while the other is occluded and the patient keeps the eyes closed. An individual with intact olfaction will be able not only to detect the smell, but also to

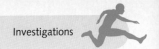

discriminate and name it. The recommended special testing bottles are rarely available when needed, and most clinicians perform preliminary assessment with nearby objects such as a coffee jar or gum. It is important to avoid using pungent odors like cleaning solutions, which would activate the trigeminal nerve. When examining patients with anosmia, it is important to look carefully for frontal lobe signs and evidence of optic nerve or chiasmal damage. More often there will be pathology in the nasal passages or sinuses.

Investigations

Unexplained anosmia may require referral for more expert otolaryngology examination if there is no suspicion of a neurologic cause. In some cases, computerized tomography or magnetic resonance imaging is justifiable to rule out a frontal tumor. Established posttraumatic anosmia requires no investigation unless there are also features to suggest a cerebrospinal fluid fistula or intracranial infection.

5. Visual Impairment

Disturbance of vision may be due to disease of the cornea, iris, ciliary body, anterior chamber, lens, vitreous humor, choroid, or retina. These pathologies are usually dealt with by the ophthalmologist and will not be discussed here. Visual impairment presenting to the neurologist usually involves a lesion in the visual pathway from the optic nerve to the occipital cortex.

The visual pathway

The visual pathway extends from the retina to the occipital cortex. The retina consists of three distinct layers (Fig. 5.1). Light falls on rods and cones, which lie in the outermost layer, above the pigmented epithelium. Rods are responsible for night vision and detection of peripheral movement. Cones are responsible for daytime and color vision. Impulses are transmitted by bipolar cells, with which the rods and cones synapse, to the ganglion cells and their unmyelinated fibers. These fibers run into the optic disc, where they become myelinated, and exit as the optic nerve. The macula is a region of the retina specialized for perception of detailed images and color. It contains the greatest concentration of cones and has no rods. The latter are more abundant in the peripheral retina.

Light from an object in, for example, the right temporal field of vision will cast an image on the temporal retina of the left eye and the nasal retina of the right eye. Light from the upper field of vision will cast an image in the lower part of the retina. Fibers from the temporal region of each retina run in the temporal half of the optic nerve, those from the nasal region of the retina, in the nasal half of the nerve; the macular fibers run centrally. At the optic chiasm, the nasal fibers from each retina cross to the opposite side while the temporal fibers continue their course ipsilaterally. Beyond the optic chiasm, the fibers on each side form the optic tract and pass posteriorly to synapse in the lateral geniculate bodies. Fibers from

the latter continue posteriorly in the internal capsule, coursing deep into the parietal (uppermost fibers) and temporal (lowermost fibers) lobes and ultimately terminating in the occipital cortex. The arterial supply to the occipital cortex is from the posterior cerebral artery. However, the middle cerebral artery supplies the tip of the occipital pole, where fibers from the macula ultimately terminate.

Visual field defects at different sites of the optic pathway are shown in Fig. 5.2. Clinical features at each of the anatomical levels shown are discussed.

Clinical features to aid lesion localization

The clinical features that aid anatomic localization of the lesion in a patient with a visual field defect are as follows.

Optic nerve lesion

Visual loss in one eye represents retinal or optic nerve dysfunction. The patient with an optic nerve lesion complains of blurred vision and, with inflammatory lesions of the nerve, of pain with eye movements on that side. On examination there is reduced visual acuity, reduction of color vision, and a central scotoma. An afferent pupillary defect and pale optic disc may be present.

Lesions of the optic nerve include:
- Optic neuritis (multiple sclerosis).
- Optic nerve meningioma or glioma.
- Giant-cell arteritis.

Optic chiasm lesion

A chiasmal lesion causes a bitemporal hemianopia due to compression of the decussating nasal fibers (Fig. 5.2[3]). Pressure from a lesion below the chiasm will involve the inferior nasal fibers first, resulting in a bitemporal superior quadrantanopia; pressure from a lesion above the chiasm will cause an inferior quadrantanopia. The patient often either

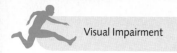
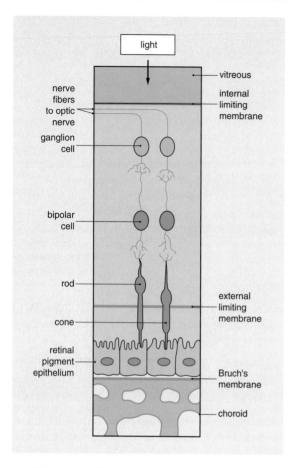

Fig. 5.1 Layers of the retina.

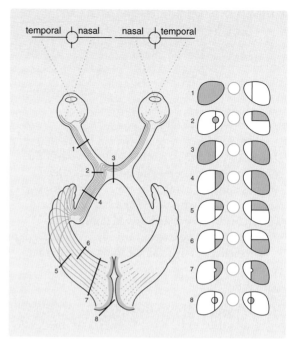

Fig. 5.2 Lesions of different parts of the visual pathway produce characteristic field defects.

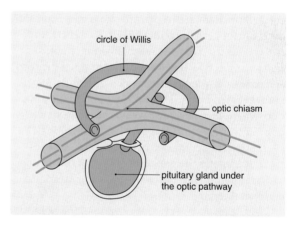

Fig. 5.3 Relation of the optic chiasm to its surrounding structures.

complains of unilateral visual disturbance or does not complain of visual problems at all but may bump into objects in either temporal field. The lesion may compress one or both optic nerves, giving rise to additional signs of an optic nerve lesion—i.e., reduced visual acuity and color vision, a central scotoma, and eventually a pale disc and afferent pupillary defect.

The relations of the optic chiasm are shown in Fig. 5.3. Double vision is uncommon but may occur if the lesion extends to involve the ocular motor nerves in the cavernous sinus.

Lesions of the optic chiasm include:

- Tumors—e.g., pituitary adenoma, meningioma, craniopharyngioma, or metastatic deposits.
- Cerebral aneurysm (note proximity of the circle of Willis).
- Granulomatous disease—tuberculosis, sarcoidosis.
- Rathke's cleft cyst.

Optic tract and optic radiation lesions

Lesions of the optic tract and optic radiation cause a contralateral homonymous hemianopia. Those involving the parietal fibers give rise to an inferior quadrantanopia and those involving the temporal lobe fibers a superior quadrantanopia ("pie in the sky"; see Fig. 5.2). The patient often attributes the problem only to the eye on the hemianopic side. If the field loss is incongruous (i.e., different in the two eyes), the lesion is more likely to be anteriorly placed (usually the optic tract); if it is congruous, it is likely to be placed more posteriorly, near the occipital cortex.

Note that lesions of the optic tract only are uncommon and usually caused by posterior extension of a pituitary tumor.

Lesions of the optic tract and optic radiation include:

• Infarction, such as a lesion of the middle cerebral artery.
• Intracerebral hemorrhage.
• Tumors.
• Trauma.
• Demyelination.

Occipital cortex lesions

Unilateral lesions of the posterior cerebral artery (e.g., embolism from the vertebrobasilar arterial tree) cause a contralateral homonymous hemianopia with sparing of the macula (Figs. 5.2[7] and 5.4), which is supplied by the middle cerebral artery.

Damage to the tip of the occipital pole involves the macular fibers and gives rise to a central homonymous hemianopic defect (see Figs. 5.2[8] and 5.4).

Bilateral occipital cortex damage (e.g., tumor, trauma, infarction) gives rise to cortical blindness characterized by visual loss throughout the field in both eyes and preserved pupillary responses. If the visual association areas are involved, patients with cortical blindness may claim that they can see when clearly they cannot—this is Anton's syndrome.

A central scotoma may be caused by:
• Retinal disease involving the macula.
• Lesions of the optic nerve.
• Damage of the occipital pole (when scotomas affect <u>both</u> eyes).

Differential diagnosis

When a patient presents with visual impairment, it is important to ascertain whether it is acute or subacute. Patients usually complain of unilateral visual disturbance. Presentation with bilateral disturbance is uncommon even if the patient has a bilateral field deficit. Papilledema is an important cause of bilateral visual impairment. Less common causes are cortical blindness and psychogenic blindness.

Acute visual impairment

The first step is to determine whether the acute visual impairment or loss is transient or persistent.

Acute transient visual impairment

Causes of acute transient visual impairment or loss include:

• Amaurosis fugax.
• Migraine with aura.
• Papilledema.
• Uhthoff's phenomenon.

Amaurosis fugax

With amaurosis fugax, the patient complains of sudden unilateral altitudinal visual loss, often described as a shutter coming down from the superior to inferior part of the visual field. This lasts several seconds or minutes, followed by complete recovery.

The most common cause is stenosis of the ipsilateral carotid artery, causing embolism into the retinal arterioles.

Migraine with aura

The visual symptoms that accompany migraine headache can consist of unformed flashes of white or,

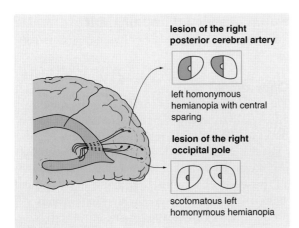

Fig. 5.4 Lesion of the occipital cortex.

lesion of the right posterior cerebral artery

left homonymous hemianopia with central sparing

lesion of the right occipital pole

scotomatous left homonymous hemianopia

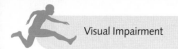

less commonly, colored lights (photopsia) or formations of dazzling zig-zag lines (fortification spectra). This visual aura can move across the visual field over 2–3 minutes, leaving scotomatous defects that are bilateral and may be homonymous. Aura symptoms generally precede the headache and last less than 60 minutes.

The diagnosis is made from a history of recurrent paroxysmal attacks with headache, photophobia, and other migrainous symptoms. Migraine aura can occur without the headache, but this is uncommon, and the differential diagnosis includes transient ischemic attacks.

Papilledema

Papilledema is swelling of the optic disc due to raised intracranial pressure. It is almost invariably bilateral. The optic nerve is covered with meninges and therefore surrounded by subarachnoid fluid. The surrounding dura mater eventually fuses with the periosteum of the orbit, and the pia and arachnoid mater with the sclera. Raised intracranial pressure in the optic nerve sheath impedes venous drainage and restricts axoplasmic flow in the nerve. Patients with moderate papilledema may have no visual symptoms. In severe cases, fleeting bilateral loss of vision (lasting a few seconds) may be experienced. On examination, visual acuity is normal, but the blind spot is enlarged, with restriction of the peripheral field of vision. The disc is swollen, with blurring of the disc margin, engorgement of the retinal veins, and flame-shaped hemorrhages on or adjacent to the disc. If the condition becomes chronic, optic atrophy and visual failure will ultimately occur.

Uhthoff's phenomenon

Uhthoff's phenomenon may cause transient visual loss in an eye that had optic neuritis. It usually lasts from minutes to 1 hour and is precipitated by heat.

Differential diagnoses of tunnel vision include:
- Papilledema.
- Glaucoma.
- Peripheral retinopathy, usually pigmentary.
- Psychogenic.
- Migraine with aura (transient tunnel vision).

Acute persistent visual impairment

Acute persistent visual impairment or loss may be due to:
- Optic or retrobulbar neuritis.
- Retinal or optic nerve ischemia.
- Arterial thromboembolism of the middle or posterior cerebral artery.

Optic and retrobulbar neuritis

Optic neuritis is inflammation of the optic nerve. If the inflammation is anterior, the disc is swollen (termed papillitis); if more posterior, it will appear normal (retrobulbar neuritis). Loss of central vision may be mild or severe. There is often a dull ache with eye movements, particularly elevation. A central scotoma, defective color vision, and an afferent pupillary defect are found. Following recovery, temporal pallor is common. The most common cause is demyelination either confined to the optic nerve or as a symptom of multiple sclerosis.

Retinal or optic nerve ischemia

Sudden monocular visual loss results from embolism into the central retinal artery or occlusion of small posterior ciliary arteries by local small-vessel disease, especially cranial arteritis.

Arterial thromboembolism of the middle or posterior cerebral artery

Arterial thromboembolic events are usually of sudden onset, although the patient may not always notice the deficit immediately. The characteristic findings are described on pp. 185–186. The history and examination should focus on cerebrovascular risk factors (e.g., ischemic heart disease, diabetes, hyperlipidemia, hypertension, atrial fibrillation).

Subacute visual impairment

Subacute visual impairment or loss may be caused by optic atrophy.

Optic atrophy

This results from damage to the nerve fibers in the visual pathway at any point between and including the ganglion cells of the retina and the lateral geniculate body. Visual loss is central but can also be peripheral. There is central disc pallor, which may also be seen with a normal large physiological cup and in the myopic eye. However, optic atrophy can be distinguished by attenuation of the retinal vessels, poor color vision, a central scotoma, and impaired afferent pupillary responses to light. Once established, the disc appearance will not return to normal despite relieving the cause; vision, however, may improve.

Causes at each level are:

- Retina—central retinal artery occlusion, retinitis pigmentosa, toxic (quinine).
- Optic nerve—optic neuritis, chronic glaucoma, long-standing papilledema, tumor, nutritional (e.g., pernicious anemia), toxic (e.g., ethyl and methyl alcohol, tobacco), hereditary, trauma.
- Chiasm and optic tract (see p. 26).

Investigation of visual symptoms

The investigation plan will be determined entirely by the differential diagnosis resulting from a careful clinical history and examination (Fig. 5.5).

Visual impairment due to ocular disease is more likely to be painful. In these cases the pain is usually localized to the eye, and there are accompanying signs in the eye. Visual impairment presenting to the neurologist is usually painless; in most cases where pain is a feature, there is headache with visual impairment. If the patient has headache and visual impairment, think of:

- Giant-cell arteritis.
- Optic neuritis.
- Glaucoma.
- Migraine (if transient).
- Severely raised intracranial pressure.
- Pituitary tumor.

Investigation plan for visual impairment	
Acute transient visual impairment	
amaurosis fugax	carotid Doppler study (cartoid artery stenosis)
migraine with aura	no investigation if the history is typical
papilledema	MRI/CT scan of the brain (raised intracranial pressure, tumor)
Acute persistent visual impairment	
optic or retrobulbar neuritis	MRI of the brain, visual evoked responses and CSF examination to look for oligoclonal bands (multiple sclerosis)
retinal or optic nerve ischemia	ESR, temporal artery biopsy (giant-cell arteritis)
arterial thromboembolism of the middle or posterior cerebral artery	fasting cholesterol and glucose, blood pressure, ECG, echocardiogram (cerebrovascular risk factors)
Subacute visual loss	
optic atrophy	MRI of the brain (tumor, multiple sclerosis), VEPs and CSF examination (multiple sclerosis), tonometry (glaucoma), vitamin B_{12} (pernicious anemia), cerebrovascular risk factors as above

Fig. 5.5 Investigation plan for visual impairment.

29

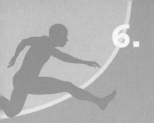

6. Disorders of the Pupils and Eye Movements

Changes of pupillary size and reactions may provide important clues to disorders of the eye itself, the second and third cranial nerves, the cervical sympathetic outflow, and the central connections of these nerves within the brainstem. Abnormalities of eye movements may also result from lesions arising in many different anatomical sites, ranging from the frontal and occipital cortex, through the basal ganglia, cerebellum, brainstem, the third, fourth, sixth and eighth cranial nerves, the neuromuscular junction, and the eye muscles themselves.

Pupil disorders

The size of the pupils is determined by the iris, which contains two groups of smooth muscle:

- The sphincter pupillae—a circular constrictor muscle innervated by the parasympathetic nervous system.
- The dilator pupillae—a radial dilator muscle innervated by the sympathetic nervous system.

Parasympathetic fibers arise in the Edinger–Westphal nucleus in the midbrain. These fibers join those of the third cranial (oculomotor) nerve and synapse in the ciliary ganglion within the orbit. The postganglionic fibers travel in the short ciliary nerves to innervate the sphincter pupillae muscle and ciliary body (Fig. 6.1).

Sympathetic fibers arise in the hypothalamus and descend uncrossed to the midbrain, pons, medulla, and lower cervical and upper thoracic spinal cord, where they synapse with the lateral horn cells. From the latter arise preganglionic fibers, which exit the cord in the anterior roots of C8 and T1 and pass through the stellate ganglion to synapse in the superior cervical ganglion. Postganglionic fibers course along the internal carotid artery, through the cavernous sinus to the long ciliary nerve, which innervates the dilator pupillae. Some fibers follow the external carotid artery and innervate Müller's muscle of the eyelid, and the blood vessels and sweat glands of the face (apart from fibers responsible for sweating of the medial aspect of the forehead, which follow the internal carotid artery).

The light reflex

When light is shone into the eye, an afferent impulse is sent from the retina to the optic nerve and tract. Fibers concerned with the light reflex synapse in the pretectal nucleus of the midbrain and then the ipsilateral and contralateral Edinger–Westphal nuclei; the rest of the fibers in the visual pathway continue on to synapse in the lateral geniculate body. The efferent pathway is from the Edinger–Westphal nucleus via the third cranial nerve to the ciliary ganglion and then to the sphincter pupillae and ciliary body on each side. Therefore, a light shone into one eye will result in equal constriction of both pupils, i.e. a direct and consensual response (Fig. 6.2).

The accommodation reflex

When looking at a near object, the eyes converge and no longer have parallel axes. The pupils constrict, and the ciliary body contracts to increase the thickness of the lens and therefore its refractive power. The descending pathway is thought to involve the parieto-occipital cortex, the Edinger–Westphal nuclei (pupillary constriction), and medial recti components of the nuclei of the third cranial nerve in the midbrain (convergence). A lesion of pupillary constrictor fibers will affect accommodation. Selective impairment of accommodation without impairment of pupillary responses to light can occur in midbrain lesions.

Differential diagnosis of pupil disorders

Anisocoria

Anisocoria is the inequality in the size of the pupils. Variable anisocoria occurs in 20% of normal people;

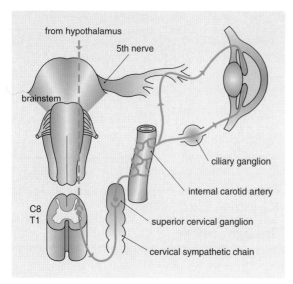

Fig. 6.1 The sympathetic pathway for pupillary dilatation.

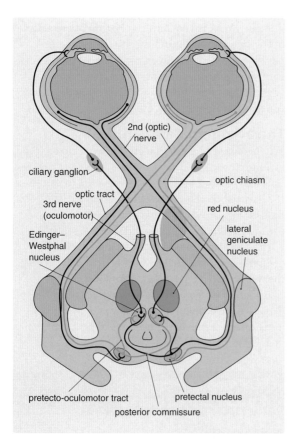

Fig. 6.2 Pathway for the light reflex and pupillary constriction.

however, it may also be a sign of central nervous system pathology.

Small constricted (miotic) pupil

Small constricted pupils may be caused by:
- Senility.
- Drugs.
- Horner's syndrome.
- Pontine lesion.
- Argyll Robertson pupils (syphilis).

Senility and drugs

When the cause is senility or drugs, both pupils are constricted, with absent or poor dilatation in the dark. Drugs to consider include opiates and pilocarpine drops used to treat chronic glaucoma.

To identify which pupil is abnormal in a patient with anisocoria, the following should be assessed:
- Pupillary responses—the abnormal pupil will have an impaired response to light, and accommodation in most cases.
- Evidence of ptosis—if there is ptosis accompanying a small pupil, look for other signs associated with a Horner's syndrome; if the ptosis is accompanied by a large pupil, look for other signs of a third nerve palsy.
- Eye movements—eye movements will be abnormal in a patient who has a third nerve palsy and therefore a fixed dilated pupil with a partial or complete ptosis.

Horner's syndrome

Interruption of the sympathetic pathway gives rise to Horner's syndrome, which is characterized by:
- Pupil constriction—the pupil reaction to light and accommodation is reduced. Dim light accentuates the anisocoria; the pupil dilates more slowly than the normal pupil.
- Ptosis (usually partial).
- Anhidrosis of the ipsilateral side of the face (lesion proximal to the carotid bifurcation) or medial side

of the forehead only (lesion distal to the bifurcation).
- Enophthalmos (a sunken eye)—this is apparent rather than actual; the eye appears sunken because of the narrowed palpebral fissure.

Horner's syndrome occurs from a lesion at any of the following levels (see Fig. 6.1):
- Brainstem—e.g., multiple sclerosis, infarction, tumor (e.g., glioma).
- Cervical cord—e.g., syringomyelia, ependymoma, tumor.
- T1 root (e.g., Pancoast tumor), cervical rib.
- Sympathetic chain—e.g., neoplastic infiltration or surgical damage in the neck involving the larynx, pharynx, thyroid; carotid artery lesions such as a dissection or trauma.

Pontine lesion
Bilateral unreactive pinpoint pupils in a comatose patient suggest a large intrapontine hemorrhage causing bilateral interruption of the sympathetic pathways. The differential is an iatrogenic cause—opiates or pilocarpine unrelated to the coma.

Argyll Robertson pupils
An Argyll Robertson pupil is small and irregular. There is no response to light, but there is a response to accommodation. The lesion is thought to be within the midbrain. Argyll Robertson pupils have characteristically been associated with syphilis. Other causes include diabetes mellitus, chronic alcoholism, multiple sclerosis, and sarcoidosis.

Large dilated (mydriatic) pupil
Large dilated pupils can be caused by:
- Lesions of the eye—e.g., damage to the iris in acute glaucoma, trauma to the sphincter muscle.
- Drugs—parasympathetic paralysis (e.g., atropine), sympathetic stimulation (e.g., epinephrine).
- Third nerve or midbrain lesions.
- Holmes–Adie pupil.
- Afferent pupillary defect.

Disorders of the iris and iatrogenic mydriasis
Local lesions of the iris may produce a dilated, usually irregular pupil. The pupillary response will depend on the degree of damage to the muscle, e.g., adhesions anteriorly to the cornea or posteriorly to the lens following inflammation or trauma, iridectomy, or tumor infiltration.

The drug history should be noted for sympathomimetics and those causing parasympathetic paralysis.

Third nerve lesions
With third nerve lesions, the pupil is dilated and both direct and consensual light responses on the affected side are absent. Look for ptosis and ophthalmoplegia caused by involvement of the levator palpebrae muscle and the superior, inferior, and medial recti and inferior oblique muscles, e.g., herniation of the temporal lobe, posterior communicating artery aneurysm, diabetes, tumors.

Midbrain lesions
Midbrain lesions involving the decussating fibers of the light reflex result in bilateral semidilated pupils without response to light. The area responsible for vertical gaze is in the midbrain, so there may also be impaired upward or downward gaze (e.g., pinealoma, infarction, demyelination, tumor deposits).

Holmes–Adie pupil
Holmes–Adie pupil is dilated and responds sluggishly, if at all, to light, but there is a better response to accommodation. It is thought to be due to degeneration of the ciliary ganglion. It usually occurs in young females and may be associated with diminished tendon reflexes.

Afferent pupillary defect
A lesion anterior to the lateral geniculate body may result in an afferent pupillary defect—the Marcus Gunn pupil. If a light is shone into the normal eye, the direct and consensual responses are normal; if a light is shone into the affected eye, the reaction to constrict is slow and may be incomplete. If the light is swung from one eye to the other (3–4 seconds on each eye), both pupils will constrict appropriately during illumination of the normal eye but both will then dilate as the light shines into the abnormal visual pathway; this results from impairment of the afferent arc of the light reflex on the abnormal side, e.g., optic neuritis, pituitary tumor.

Changes in pupil size and causes are shown in Fig. 6.3.

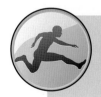
Pupil responses are normal in lesions of the optic radiation and occipital cortex.

unilateral (dilated)			reaction to light (direct)	associated signs
third nerve palsy			none	ptosis (partial or complete), external ophthalmoplegia
Holmes–Adie syndrome			slow	better response to accommodation, lower limb hyporeflexia
Marcus Gunn pupil			slow and incomplete	normal consensual response, optic atrophy, central scotoma, impaired color vision
local lesion of the iris			variable depending on extent of local damage	irregular pupil
unilateral (constricted)				
Horner's syndrome			reduced dilatation to shade	ptosis (partial), ipsilateral facial anhidrosis, "enophthalmos"
bilateral (dilated)				
midbrain lesion			none	mid-position pupils; impaired vertical gaze
iatrogenic—atropine, tricyclic antidepressants			none or reduced	
bilateral (constricted)				
senile			none or reduced	
iatrogenic—opiates, pilocarpine drops			none or reduced	
pontine lesion			none	pin-point pupils, coma, Cheyne–Stokes respiration
Argyll Robertson pupil			none	irregular pupils, normal accommodation, poorly reactive to light

Fig. 6.3 Pupil abnormalities.

Disorders of eye movements

Binocular vision allows light from an object to fall onto corresponding parts of each retina so that a single image is registered. If there is impaired movement of one eye, the image will be projected onto the macula in the normal eye and to one side of the macula in the affected eye; two images of the same object are then perceived by the higher centers of the brain.

The synchronous movements of the eyes is termed conjugate gaze. Movements of the eyes are affected by three pairs of extraocular muscles:
- The superior and inferior recti.
- The medial and lateral recti.
- The superior and inferior oblique.

All are innervated by the third cranial nerve apart from the superior oblique (innervated by the fourth cranial nerve) and lateral rectus (innervated by the sixth cranial nerve). The function of each muscle is summarized in Fig. 6.4.

Conjugate gaze

Eye movements are initiated from the ipsilateral occipital cortex or from the contralateral frontal cortex (Fig. 6.5). The former pathway is responsible for slow smooth pursuit movements used to maintain fixation of a moving image. The latter pathway is responsible for rapid saccadic movements which enable fixation of new images. Both pathways ultimately converge on the pontine center for horizontal gaze, the paramedian pontine reticular formation (PPRF), and to the midbrain for vertical gaze. From the PPRF there are connections to the sixth nerve nucleus, supplying the ipsilateral lateral rectus muscle, and to the third nerve nucleus, via the medial longitudinal fasciculus, supplying the contralateral medial rectus muscle. Vestibular and cerebellar influences are important for modulating eye movements.

Strabismus (lazy eye)

Misalignment of the visual axes gives rise to a strabismus; light from an image falls on

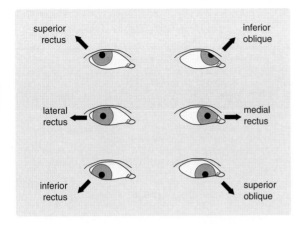

superior rectus

inferior oblique

lateral rectus

medial rectus

inferior rectus

superior oblique

Fig. 6.4 Muscles responsible for eye movements.

noncorresponding parts of the retina. Binocular vision is established by the age of 6 months. Everyone has some tendency to misalign the visual axes; however, this is overcome by mechanisms of fusion. This ensures that light from an image falls onto corresponding parts of the retina so that a single image is registered by the brain. If this does not happen, a strabismus will occur. In adulthood, the strabismus is accompanied by diplopia. When strabismus occurs in early childhood, one of the two images is suppressed by the brain so that diplopia does not occur. The eye sits in its abnormal position, drifting either outward, a divergent strabismus (exotropia), or inward, a convergent strabismus

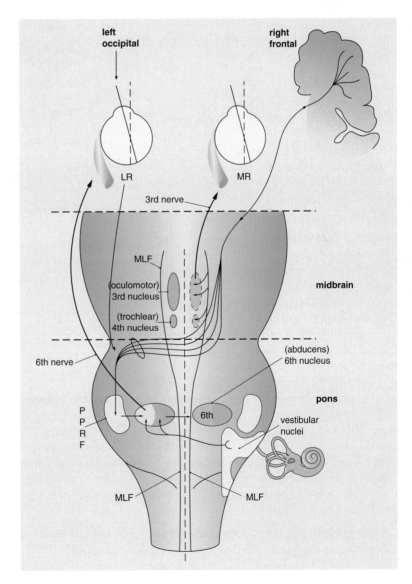

Fig. 6.5 The pathways involved in producing conjugate gaze. (LR, lateral rectus; MR, medial rectus; MLF, medial longitudinal fasciculus; PPRF, paramedian pontine reticular formation).

(esotropia). This suppression of one image interferes with the development of normal vision in that eye. If this persists beyond the age of 6 years, an amblyopic (lazy) eye develops.

Monocular diplopia

Monocular diplopia is double vision that occurs in one eye when the other eye is covered. It is due to a lesion of the eye itself. The most common causes are cataracts and corneal scarring; the alternative is a nonorganic cause.

Binocular diplopia

Binocular diplopia occurs when there is failure of established binocular vision. Misalignment of the visual axes may result from paralysis of the extraocular muscles or restriction of their normal movements by mechanical factors. The double vision resolves when either eye is covered.

Causes of diplopia

Causes of diplopia include:

- Lesions of third, fourth and/or sixth cranial nerves.
- Brainstem lesions affecting the nuclei of the third, fourth, and sixth nerves, or their connections.
- Lesions of the neuromuscular junction or muscle.
- Mechanical lesions displacing the globe within the orbit.

Lesions of third (oculomotor) nucleus and nerve

The nucleus of the third cranial nerve is situated in the midbrain. It consists of a motor nucleus for the ocular motor muscles, and the Edinger–Westphal nucleus for pupillary constriction. The nerve emerges from the midbrain and passes near to the posterior communicating artery to enter the cavernous sinus. It enters the orbit through the superior orbital fissure to supply the eyelid, the inferior oblique and superior, inferior, and medial recti muscles, and, via a parasympathetic branch, the pupil and ciliary body.

With compressive lesions of the third nerve (e.g., aneurysms, herniation of the temporal lobe), the superficially located pupillary constrictor fibers are affected early. In contrast, in diabetes there is infarction of the core of the nerve and the more superficial fibers may be unaffected, thus sparing the pupillary responses (Fig. 6.6).

Lesions of fourth (trochlear) nucleus and nerve

The nucleus of the fourth cranial nerve arises in the midbrain; fibers from here decussate and the nerve

3rd (oculomotor) cranial nerve lesions
3rd nerve and nucleus lesions give rise to:
diplopia in all directions of gaze
lateral deviation of the eye
ptosis (partial or full)
a dilated pupil unresponsive to light and accommodation
3rd nerve lesions
posterior communicating artery aneurysm
cavernous sinus thrombosis
lesions of the superior orbital fissure (malignant infiltration)
diabetes
Midbrain lesions affecting the 3rd nucleus
infarction
demyelination
glioma
metastatic deposits
Look for:
a contralateral hemiplegia
ipsilateral limb ataxia
coarse red nuclear tremor (involvement of cerebellar and red nuclear fibers)
Patient looking forward
Patient looking in the direction of the arrow

Fig. 6.6 Third cranial nerve lesions.

emerges on the dorsum of the brainstem. The trochlear nerve is the only cranial nerve that emerges from the posterior aspect of the brainstem. It has a long intracranial course and eventually traverses the cavernous sinus with the third, sixth, and ophthalmic and maxillary branches of the trigeminal (fifth) nerve, entering the orbit through the superior orbital fissure to supply the superior oblique muscle (Fig. 6.7).

Lesions of sixth (abducens) nucleus and nerve

The nucleus of the sixth cranial nerve lies in the floor of the fourth ventricle in the lower pons, circled by the seventh nerve. The nerve ascends the brainstem, passes over the tip of the petrous temporal bone, and enters the cavernous sinus. It enters the orbit through the superior orbital fissure to supply the lateral rectus muscle (Fig. 6.8).

Lesions of the brainstem

Pathology involving the brainstem may involve one or more of the third, fourth, and sixth ocular motor

4th (trochlear) cranial nerve lesions	6th (abducens) cranial nerve lesions

4th nerve and nucleus lesions give rise to paralysis of the superior oblique muscle:
vertical and oblique diplopia on looking down and inwards
the eye sits rotated slightly outwards and upwards (extorsion)
the patient tries to compensate by tilting the head away from
the affected eye (head tilt to opposite shoulder)

6th nerve and nucleus lesions give rise to paralysis of the lateral rectus muscle:
horizontal diplopia maximal on lateral gaze to the side
of the lesion

4th nerve lesions
isolated 4th nerve lesions are rare and usually due to diabetes
(ischemic infarction of the nerve) or trauma
lesions of the cavernous sinus and superior orbital fissure
will involve the 3rd and 6th nerves, and branches of the 5th nerve

6th nerve lesions
Gradenigo's syndrome—due to infection of the petrous
temporal bone (usually affects CNV and VI)
cavernous sinus thrombosis
fracture or malignant infiltration (nasopharyngeal
carcinoma) of the skull base
lesions of the superior orbital fissure

4th nucleus lesions
same as for the third nucleus (see Fig. 6.6)

6th nucleus lesions
same as for the 3rd and 4th nucleus (see Fig. 6.6)

Look for:
contralateral hemiplegia
ipsilateral weakness of the upper and lower face (7th nerve
fibers hooking around the 6th nucleus)

Patient looking forward

Patient looking forward

Patient looking in the direction of the arrow

Patient looking in the direction of the arrow

Fig. 6.7 Fourth cranial nerve lesions. Note that the weakness of the superior oblique muscle is contralateral to the side of the fourth nucleus lesion.

Fig. 6.8 Sixth cranial nerve lesions. Note, in cases of raised intracranial pressure, due to its long course, the sixth nerve may become stretched as it passes over the tip of the petrous temporal bone, giving rise to a sixth nerve palsy—this is a false localizing sign.

nuclei, as detailed individually (see Figs. 6.6, 6.7 and 6.8). The blood supply to these nuclei is from the vertebrobasilar arterial tree, so occlusive vascular disease may cause transient or permanent diplopia due to involvement of all the ocular motor nuclei.

Vascular or demyelinating disease of the medial longitudinal fasciculus gives rise to diplopia due to an internuclear ophthalmoplegia (see pp. 144–145).

Disorders of the neuromuscular junction
Diplopia and ptosis are common presenting features of Myasthenia Gravis; both are fatiguable. A positive tensilon test is diagnostic but is not always present.

Disorders of muscle
Thyroid myopathy most frequently involves the medial and inferior recti.

Progressive ocular myopathy is a muscular dystrophy that causes diplopia from weakness of the extraocular muscles, ptosis, and weakness of the facial and limb-girdle muscles.

If diplopia is due to a third, fourth, <u>and</u> sixth nerve palsy, think of a lesion of the:
- Brainstem.
- Cavernous sinus.
- Superior orbital fissure.

If examination does not reveal the diplopia to be consistent with defined weakness of one or more of the extraocular muscles (see Fig. 6.4, p. 35), consider Myasthenia Gravis, look for proptosis and a mechanical etiology, or consider a nonorganic cause.

Orbital lesions

Displacement of the globe will result in diplopia. Causes include:

- Retro-orbital arteriovenous malformations and tumor deposits—look for proptosis.
- A "blow-out" fracture of the orbit—fracture of the floor of the orbit with herniation of the soft tissues into the maxillary sinus; look for enophthalmos (sunken eye), restricted eye movements, and loss of sensation in the area supplied by the inferior orbital nerve.

Abnormalities of conjugate gaze
Horizontal gaze palsy

Horizontal gaze palsy is caused by a lesion in the frontal cortex or pons; therefore, hemiparesis is usually present. The direction of limitation of the conjugate gaze will depend on the site of the lesion. The direction of deviation of the eye relative to the neurological deficit will aid lesion localization:

- Eyes deviate away from the hemiparetic side (eyes looking at the "good" side)—frontal lobe lesion contralateral to the hemiparesis.
- Eyes deviate toward the hemiparetic side—pontine lesion contralateral to the hemiparesis.

During a focal seizure, the converse pattern is seen; i.e., in a frontal lobe seizure the eyes deviate away from the side of the lesion.

Internuclear ophthalmoplegia

A lesion of the medial longitudinal fasciculus results in an internuclear ophthalmoplegia. Internuclear ophthalmoplegia is characterized by paresis of the ipsilateral medial rectus muscle. With attempted horizontal gaze to one side, the adducting eye (the eye moving toward the nose) fails to move past midline, and the abducting eye moves fully outward but develops coarse nystagmus. Accommodation will still be intact, unless the lesion is in the medial longitudinal fasciculus.

The most common causes are demyelination and vascular lesions. Bilateral lesions are almost pathognomonic of demyelination (Fig. 6.9).

One-and-a-half syndrome

With a lower pontine lesion, the patient may have a sixth nerve plasy and bilateral internuclear ophthalmoplegia. One eye is paralyzed for all horizontal movements; the other eye can make only abducting movements with coarse nystagmus.

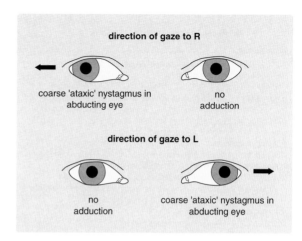

Fig. 6.9 Bilateral internuclear ophthalmoplegia.

Nystagmus

Nystagmus is abnormal involuntary oscillatory movements of the eye. There are two types:

- Jerk nystagmus is characterized by a slow component and a fast corrective component in the opposite direction. The direction of the nystagmus is described in terms of the direction of the fast component.
- Pendular nystagmus is characterized by equal oscillations in both directions.

Nystagmus can be subdivided into central and peripheral pathways. The central pathways involve the vestibular nuclei in the brainstem and their connections. Nystagmus from pure cerebellar disease is rare and usually involves the brainstem connections. The peripheral pathways include the vestibular nerve and labyrinth.

It is first important to distinguish nonpathologic from pathologic nystagmus.

Nonpathologic nystagmus
Nystagmoid jerks

Fine nystagmus can be seen:

- If eye movements are tested too fast.
- At the extremes of lateral gaze beyond the range of binocular vision.

Optokinetic nystagmus

Normally, when watching a moving object (e.g., trees from a moving train or vertical stripes on a rotating drum), nystagmoid jerks occurs. The slow component represents normal pursuit movements to the limit of conjugate gaze; the fast component in the opposite direction represents rapid saccadic movements with subsequent fixation on a new object entering the field of view. Optokinetic nystagmus (OKN) is interrupted in lesions of the parietal cortex and its connections to the brainstem centers involved in conjugate gaze. If the above-mentioned rotating drum is rotated towards the side of the lesion, OKN is lost or reduced; if rotated in the opposite direction, OKN is normal. OKN is normal in disorders of the peripheral vestibular system and in nonorganic blindness (i.e., psychogenic blindness).

Pendular nystagmus due to visual impairment

An acquired pendular nystagmus occurs in patients with marked visual impairment or loss in early life (e.g., albinism, congenital cataracts). The nystagmus is always in the horizontal plane whether the eye movements are vertical or horizontal. At the extremes of gaze, jerk nystagmus may be seen.

Congenital nystagmus

Congenital nystagmus is a pendular nystagmus present in all positions of gaze, often including the resting position. The condition is present from birth and has an autosomal dominant inheritance. The patient is unaware of the movement due to synchronized oscillations of the head in the opposite direction, which steady the image.

Central nystagmus
Lesions of the brainstem vestibular nuclei

Vertical nystagmus occurs in lesions of the pons and medulla. Note that vertigo is uncommon. There are two types of vertical nystagmus:

- Upbeat nystagmus is seen in patients with, for example, multiple sclerosis, vascular disorders, or tumors.

- Downbeat nystagmus is characteristic of lesions at the foramen magnum (e.g., Arnold–Chiari malformation).

Both types are seen in Wernicke's disease.

In comatose patients with extensive pontine lesions and absent horizontal eye movements, "ocular bobbing" may be seen—fast jerk movements downward, followed by a slow drift upward.

Ataxic nystagmus

Ataxic nystagmus occurs in internuclear ophthalmoplegia (see pp. 144–145).

Lesions of the vestibular connections of the cerebellum

In lesions of the vestibular connections of the cerebellum, the nystagmus is horizontal and coarse, with the fast phase towards the side of the lesion.

Peripheral nystagmus

Vertigo is a common feature with peripheral nystagmus. This is usually rotational, but can be to-and-fro. The rotation is away from the side of the lesion.

Nystagmus is horizontal, with the fast phase away from the side of the lesion in all positions of gaze. There may be unsteadiness of gait towards the side of lesion, deafness and tinnitus on the affected side, and nausea and vomiting accompanying the vertigo.

Causes include:

- Labyrinthine disease (common)—benign positional vertigo, Ménière's disease, infection, trauma.
- Vestibular nerve lesion (rare)—acoustic neuroma, aminoglycoside toxicity, herpes zoster infection.

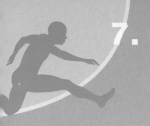

7. Facial Sensory Loss and Weakness

Facial sensory disturbance may result from disorders affecting the trigeminal (fifth cranial) nerve or its central connections within the brainstem (and high cervical cord), thalamus, internal capsule, and cerebral sensory cortex. The upper cervical nerve roots (C2, C3) also subserve sensation over a small part of the face, along the lower jaw.

Facial weakness may result from lesions involving the seventh cranial nerve and its central connections in the brainstem, internal capsule, and motor cortex, or from disease of the neuromuscular junction (myasthenia) or of muscle itself (myopathies, dystrophies).

The trigeminal nerve

The fifth cranial nerve is a mixed motor and sensory nerve. It arises from the inferolateral aspect of the pons and has a large sensory root and a small motor root.

From the pons, the sensory root pierces the dura mater to join the gasserian (trigeminal) ganglion; the ganglion cells of the sensory root all lie in the gasserian ganglion. The latter lies at the apex of the petrous temporal bone. The peripheral branches of the ganglion are in three divisions:

- Ophthalmic branch (V_1)—this traverses the lateral wall of the cavernous sinus and enters the orbit through the superior orbital fissure. Its cutaneous distribution is shown in Fig. 7.1; it also supplies the cornea, mucosa of the nasal cavity and frontal sinuses, dura mater of the falx, and the superior surface of the tentorium.
- Maxillary branch (V_2)—this traverses the lower lateral wall of the cavernous sinus and exits the skull in the foramen rotundum. It enters the floor of the orbit via the inferior orbital fissure. In addition to supplying the skin (see Fig. 7.1), it supplies the floor of the middle cranial fossa, the upper teeth and gums, and the adjacent palate.

It contributes secretory fibers to the lacrimal gland.
- Mandibular branch (V_3)—this carries the motor component of the nerve. It exits the skull via the foramen ovale. Its sensory supply is to the skin (see Fig. 7.1), mucosa of the cheek, lower lip, jaw, incisor and canine teeth, floor of the mouth, lower gums, anterior two-thirds of the tongue, and the dura mater above the tentorium.

The proximal axons of the ganglion cells in the sensory root divide in the pons into short ascending and long descending branches. The former carry light-touch and deep-pressure, and proprioceptive information, and terminate in the main sensory and mesencephalic nuclei, respectively. The long descending fibers form the spinal trigeminal tract and carry information about pain and temperature. The nucleus of the spinal trigeminal tract extends from the junction of the pons and medulla to C2 of the spinal cord. Fibers from the aforementioned nuclei cross to the opposite side and ascend to the thalamus (the trigemino-thalamic tract) and ultimately synapse in the sensory cortex (Fig. 7.2).

The motor nucleus of the fifth nerve is situated in the midpons. The fibers from the motor root pass below the gasserian ganglion and join the sensory fibers in the mandibular nerve. These motor fibers innervate the muscles of mastication.

Differential diagnosis of facial sensory loss

Because of its wide anatomic distribution, complete motor and sensory lesions of the fifth nerve are uncommon; partial damage is more often observed, particularly of the sensory component. On examination look for:
- Sensory deficit in the distribution of the branch(es) of the fifth nerve—loss of the corneal

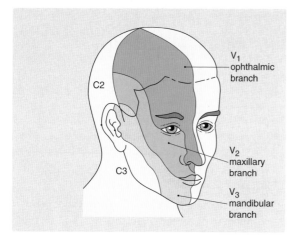

Fig. 7.1 The cutaneous distribution of the trigeminal nerve. Note that the upper cervical dermatomes (C3) extend onto the face, above the angle of the jaw.

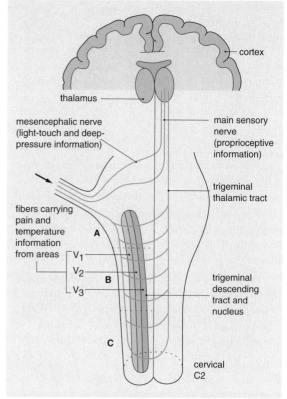

Fig. 7.2 Anatomy of the trigeminal sensory pathways.

reflex is an early sign of damage to the ophthalmic branch. Note, lesions of the lower pons, medulla, or upper cervical cord produce dissociated sensory loss of pain and temperature in an "onion skin" distribution, sparing the center of the face (territory A in Fig. 7.3) until last.

- Motor involvement—this may be manifested by weakness of the muscles of mastication, and deviation of the jaw towards the side of the lesion because of weakness of the pterygoid muscles.
- The jaw jerk (a trigeminal pontine reflex)—this is brisk in upper motor neuron lesions above the motor nucleus of the fifth nerve.

Facial sensory loss can be caused by a lesion anywhere in the pathway involving the fifth nerve and its connections. The site of the lesion can be determined by localizing the site of accompanying signs as described below. (Note, the terms ipsilateral and contralateral are relative to the side of the facial sensory loss.)

A supranuclear lesion is contralateral to the facial sensory loss. Lesions at all other sites decribed below are ipsilateral to the facial sensory loss.

Supranuclear lesions

In patients with a supranuclear lesion look for:
- Ipsilateral "pyramidal" weakness.
- Ipsilateral lower facial weakness.

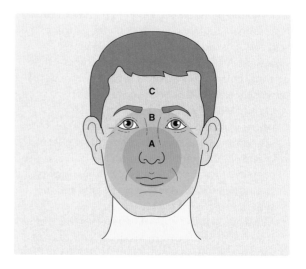

Fig. 7.3 Low pontine, medullary, and cervical lesions produce an "onion skin" distribution of pinprick (pain) and temperature loss.

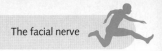

Causes of a supranuclear lesion include:
- Infarction.
- Demyelination.
- Neoplasia (glioma, metastatic deposits).

Brainstem lesions

In patients with a brainstem lesion look for:
- Contralateral corticospinal tract weakness.
- Ipsilateral cranial nerve lesions (depending on which adjacent cranial nuclei are involved).
- Lesions of the pons—conjugate gaze palsies.
- Lesions of the lower pons, medulla or upper cervical cord—dissociated sensory loss due to involvement of the trigeminal spinal tract and/or nucleus; there is contralateral loss of pain and temperature ("onion skin" distribution) with preservation of light touch, vibration, and two-point discrimination.

Causes of a brainstem lesion include:
- Infarction.
- Syringobulbia.
- Demyelination.
- Neoplasia (glioma, metastatic disease).

Cerebellopontine angle lesions

In patients with a lesion of the cerebellopontine angle look for:
- Contralateral "pyramidal" weakness.
- Damage of the ipsilateral seventh and eighth cranial nerves; late involvement of the sixth, ninth and tenth nerves.
- Ipsilateral cerebellar signs in the limbs.

Causes of a cerebellopontine angle lesion include:
- Acoustic neuroma.
- Meningioma.
- Metastatic deposits.
- Tuberculosis.
- Sarcoidosis.

Cavernous sinus lesions

In patients with a lesion of the cavernous sinus look for palsies of the third, fourth, and sixth cranial nerves, all of which also traverse the cavernous sinus. The ophthalmic branch and occasionally the maxillary branch of the fifth nerve are involved.
Causes of a cavernous sinus lesion include:
- Thrombosis of the cavernous sinus.
- Aneurysm of the intracavernous internal carotid artery.

- Extension of a pituitary tumor or metastatic infiltration.
- Benign granulomatous reactions (steroid-responsive).

Lesions of the apex of the petrous temporal bone

Pathology here may involve the gasserian ganglion and the trigeminal root.

Causes of a lesion of the apex of the petrous temporal bone include:
- Gradenigo's syndrome (which is associated with a sixth nerve palsy—from middle ear infection).
- Osteomyelitis.
- Tumors of the petrous bone.

Lesions of the trigeminal root, ganglion, and peripheral branches of the nerve

These lesions include:
- Herpes zoster—this manifests as a vesicular rash in the cutaneous distribution of the nerve.
- Skull fractures affecting the superficial branches of the trigeminal nerve (cutaneous deficit) or at the skull base (additional cranial nerve palsies).
- Neoplastic infiltration or compression—tumors of the sinuses, cholesteatoma, fifth nerve neuroma, nasopharyngeal carcinoma at the skull base, lesion of the superior orbital fissure (third, fourth and sixth nerve palsies).
- Granulomatous disease—tuberculosis, sarcoidosis.
- Vasculitis—systemic lupus erythematosus, Sjögren's syndrome.
- Trigeminal neuralgia.

The facial nerve

The seventh cranial nerve is composed of the facial nerve, which innervates the muscles of facial expression, and the stapedius, the nervus intermedius, which carries taste fibers from the anterior two-thirds of the tongue (via the chorda tympani) and parasympathetic secretomotor fibers to the salivary glands. The nucleus of the facial nerve lies in the lateral pons; its intrapontine fibers hook around the nucleus of the sixth nerve (abducens) before emerging from the pons. It enters the internal auditory meatus with the nervus intermedius and the eighth nerve, coursing the facial canal in the petrous temporal bone, angling sharply thereafter to the geniculate ganglion. Distal to the ganglion it gives off several branches—the greater superficial petrosal to the lacrimal gland, a small branch to the stapedius, and the chorda tympani, which joins a branch of the mandibular division of the fifth nerve, together conveying taste and sensation to the anterior two-thirds of the tongue. Thereafter the nerve exits the skull through the stylomastoid foramen and enters the parotid gland, where it divides into branches that supply the muscles of facial expression (Fig. 7.4).

Supranuclear fibers are from the contralateral cerebral cortex and corticobulbar tracts. The lower facial muscles have input from the contralateral hemisphere only; the upper muscles from both. Consequently, a supranuclear (upper motor neuron) lesion will cause contralateral weakness of only the lower facial muscles since the upper facial muscles have an additional supply from the intact ipsilateral supranuclear connections. In contrast, a lower motor neuron lesion will cause ipsilateral weakness involving both the upper and lower facial muscles.

Examination and differential diagnosis of facial weakness

Facial weakness arises from a lesion in the pathway of the seventh cranial nerve and its connections (including the neuromuscular junction and muscle). The first step is to distinguish the type of weakness, i.e., is it of upper or lower motor neuron type? Lesions of the neuromuscular junction and muscle cause weakness of the upper and lower face as in a lower motor neuron lesion, but this is bilateral and usually symmetrical.

Investigation of facial numbness and weakness

Because of the huge range of conditions affecting the trigeminal and facial nerves and their connections, investigations should be selected on the basis of a carefully considered clinical differential diagnosis (Fig. 7.5).

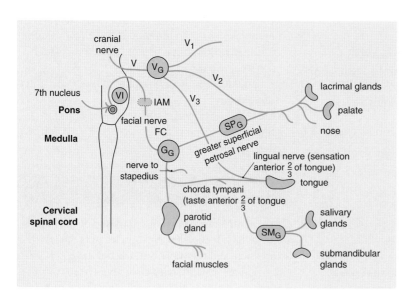

Fig. 7.4 The anatomy of the facial nerve. (V$_G$, gasserian ganglion; G$_G$ geniculate ganglion; SP$_G$, sphenopalatine ganglion; SM$_G$, submandibular ganglion; IAM, internal auditory meatus; FC, facial canal in the petrous temporal bone.)

Differential diagnosis of facial weakness	
Unilateral upper motor neuron facial weakness	**Unilateral weakness of the lower face** unilateral weakness of the lower face is due to a contralateral supranuclear (upper motor neuron) lesion; look for ipsilateral "pyramidal" signs in the limbs; the lesion may be caused by infarction, neoplastic infiltration, or demyelination
Bilateral upper motor neuron facial weakness	**Bilateral weakness of the lower face** bilateral lower facial weakness does not really occur; bilateral upper motor neuron lesions also affect the forehead
Unilateral lower motor neuron facial weakness	**Unilateral weakness of the upper and lower face** unilateral weakness of the upper and lower face is due to disorder of the nucleus of the 7th nerve, the geniculate ganglion, or the peripheral nerve; additional clinical features aid lesion localization; lesions may occur at the following sites: • pons—features include ipsilateral 6th nerve lesion and contralateral "pyramidal" weakness (recall that the intrapontine fibers hook around the nucleus of the 6th nerve); e.g., infarction, demyelination, tumor deposits • cerebellopontine angle—as for facial sensory loss • facial canal—features include hyperacusis (involvement of the stapedius, which normally dampens sound) and loss of taste in the anterior two-thirds of the tongue (involvement of the chorda tympani); e.g., middle ear infection, Bell's palsy, tumor deposits, fracture of the skull base, lyme disease • geniculate ganglion—e.g., herpes zoster infection of the ganglion; look for pain and vesicles in the auditory canal • peripheral branches of the nerve—e.g., parotid gland lesions (tumor, infection, sarcoidosis-uveoparotid fever), trauma
Bilateral lower motor neuron facial weakness	**Bilateral weakness of the upper and lower face** If a patient presents with bilateral upper and lower facial weakness (i.e., bilateral lower motor neuron facial weakness), the following differential diagnoses should be borne in mind: • Guillain Barré syndrome • sarcoidosis • bilateral Bell's palsy • myasthenia gravis • myopathies—dystrophia myotonica, facio-scapulo-humeral dystrophy • motor neuron disease • lyme disease note that disorders of the neuromuscular junction and muscle cause bilateral facial weakness.

Fig. 7.5 Possible investigations for patients presenting with facial weakness and/or numbness.

45

8. Deafness and Tinnitus

Deafness and tinnitus usually result from end-organ (cochlear) disease in the ear, and these are not often the main presenting symptoms of a neurologic disorder. However, acoustic neuroma is a rare but important "neurologic" cause of deafness and the eighth (vestibulocochlear) cranial nerve may also be involved by other conditions affecting the brainstem or multiple cranial nerves.

The eighth cranial nerve is comprised of the cochlear nerve, which subserves hearing, and the vestibular nerve, which is concerned with maintenance of balance (Fig. 8.1). Deafness and tinnitus arise from damage to the auditory apparatus and its central connections via the eighth nerve.

The auditory system

Sound waves are channelled through the external auditory meatus to the tympanic membrane and thence by the auditory ossicles to the perilymph of the cochlea (Fig. 8.1). The vibration thus set up in the perilymph is transduced into nerve impulses by the end organ of hearing, the spiral organ of Corti. The afferent impulses are transmitted by the cochlear nerve, which synapses in the cochlear nuclei in the lower pons (Fig. 8.2).

From the cochlear nuclei there are bilateral supranuclear connections to the superior olivary nuclei on each side. Fibers from the superior olive project to the inferior colliculus, the medial geniculate nucleus of the thalamus, and ultimately through the internal capsule to the auditory cortex in the superior temporal gyrus (Heschl's gyrus).

Differential diagnosis of deafness

There are two types of deafness:
- Conductive—failure of transmission of sound from the outer or middle ear to the cochlea.
- Sensorineural—due to disease of the cochlea, cochlear nerve, and cochlear nuclei and their supranuclear connections.

Clinically, conductive and sensorineural deafness can be distinguished by the Rinne and Weber tests for hearing.

Rinne's test
The base of a vibrating 128-, 256-, or 512-Hz tuning fork is held first against the mastoid process, and then, when the tone has disappeared, about 2.5 cm from the external auditory meatus. The transmission of sound through the outer and middle ear to the cochlea is better than that through bone to the cochlea (thus bypassing the middle ear apparatus). Normally, therefore, air conduction is better than bone conduction.

In conductive deafness, this ability is impaired due to disease of the outer or middle ear and bone conduction is better than air conduction. In sensorineural deafness, both sound conduction and bone conduction are diminished, but air conduction remains better than bone conduction.

Weber's test
When a vibrating tuning fork is placed in the middle of the forehead, sound is normally heard equally in both ears. In conductive deafness, the sound localizes to the affected ear (due to lack of competitive sounds that would normally be heard on that side). By contrast, in sensorineural deafness, the sound lateralizes to the normal ear.

Conductive deafness
In conductive deafness, there is impaired perception of low-pitched sounds.
Conductive deafness can be caused by:
- Disorders of the outer ear—these are usually due to the normal occurrence of wax.
- Disorders of the middle ear—otitis media, cholesteatoma, otosclerosis, rupture of the tympanic membrane.

Sensorineural deafness
In sensorineural deafness, there is impaired perception of high-pitched sounds. Sensorineural deafness can be caused by a variety of disorders, as listed below.

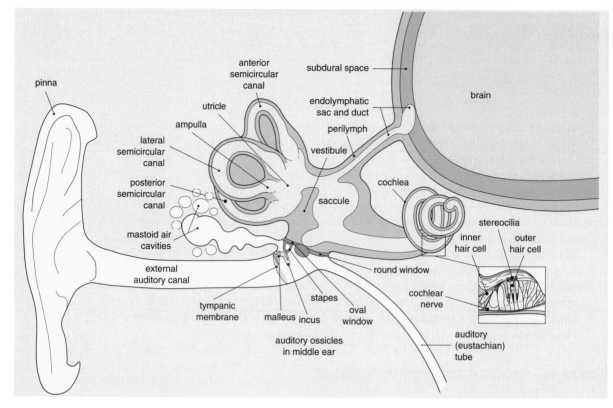

Fig. 8.1 Components of the outer, middle, and inner ear.

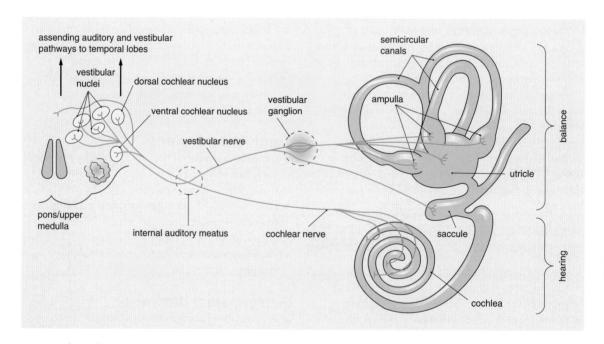

Fig. 8.2 The auditory and vestibular system.

Disorders of the cochlea

Disorders of the cochlea include:

- Congenital disorders—from rubella or syphilis in the pregnant mother.
- Infection—purulent meningitis, spread of infection from the middle to the inner ear, mumps.
- Drugs—aminoglycosides, salicylates, quinine. (Deafness is transient with the latter two.)
- Presbycusis—neuronal degeneration in the elderly causing high-frequency hearing loss.
- Noise-induced disorders—high-frequency hearing loss from, for example, gun blasts.
- Ménière's disease—vertigo and variable tinnitus and deafness.

Disorders of the cochlear nerve

Disorders of the cochlear nerve include:

- Lesions of the cerebellopontine angle (e.g., acoustic neuroma, other tumors, granulomatous disease).

 Conductive or sensorineural deafness is a feature of many inherited syndromes.

Disorders of the brainstem

Disorders of the brainstem include:

- Multiple sclerosis—plaques of demyelination involving the cochlear nuclei.
- Infarction.
- Neoplastic infiltration.

Disorders of the supranuclear connections

Unilateral lesions of the supranuclear pathways will not cause deafness as the cochlear nuclei on each side have bilateral connections projecting to the temporal cortices.

Auditory hallucinations can occur as part of temporal lobe seizures.

Investigations

There are several audiometric procedures that can distinguish deafness caused by cochlear lesions from those caused by lesions of the eighth nerve. Auditory evoked potentials test the integrity of the pathway from the cochlea to the auditory cortex in the temporal lobe. This test does not need the cooperation of the patient; i.e., it can be done in a comatose patient.

Differential diagnosis of tinnitus

Tinnitus is the sensation of ringing, buzzing, hissing, chirping, or whistling in the ear. It is a manifestation of disease of the middle ear, inner ear, or cochlear component of the eighth nerve, and is usually accompanied by some degree of deafness; examples of etiologies are summarized in Fig. 8.3. Conductive deafness is associated with low-pitched tinnitus, and sensorineural deafness with high-pitched tinnitus (except Ménière's disease, where the tinnitus is low-pitched). Vibratory mechanical noises in the head can be mistaken for tinnitus. The most common is a bruit from turbulent blood flow in the great vessels of the neck (as may occur in a febrile or anemic state); other sources include an arteriovenous malformation or carotid artery stenosis. In these situations, the noise heard is in time with the pulse.

Causes of deafness and tinnitus	
Site of damage	Cause
outer ear	wax
middle ear	trauma, e.g., fracture of temporal bone infection, e.g., suppurative otitis media, otosclerosis
cochlea	age (presbyacusis) infection, e.g., purulent meningitis noise induced drugs, e.g., aminoglycosides Ménière's disease
8th nerve	lesions of the cerebellopontine angle, e.g., acoustic neuroma basal meningitis, e.g., TB, sarcoid, malignant infiltration
brainstem (rare)	multiple sclerosis neoplasia infarction
cerebral hemisphere (rare)	bilateral lesions of the temporal lobes, e.g., infarction, neoplasia

Fig. 8.3 Causes of deafness and tinnitus.

9. Dizziness and Vertigo

Dizziness is a very common symptom. The term is nonspecific and may be used by patients to describe not only vertigo but also feelings of faintness, disorientation, drowsiness, visual disturbance, or even unsteadiness in the legs. It is important to separate all of these from the phenomenon of vertigo, which is best defined as an illusion or hallucination of movement. This perceived movement may be rotational ("true" vertigo), but often it has a swaying, rocking, or heaving quality. All of these feelings of movement are a clear indication of a disorder of the vestibular system, namely the end organs in the inner ear or their central connections in the brainstem and temporal lobe. The vestibular apparatus and brainstem nuclei are shown in Figs. 8.1 and 8.2.

The vestibular system

Contribution from the vestibular, visual, and proprioceptive systems is required to maintain balance. The labyrinth is the vestibular apparatus that lies in the inner ear on each side. It consists of the utricle, saccule, and semicircular canals. There are three semicircular canals (lateral, anterior, and posterior), each positioned perpendicularly with respect to one another. They respond to rotational acceleration of the head. The utricle and saccule respond to linear acceleration, including gravity. Afferent information from the labyrinth is relayed by the vestibular component of eighth cranial nerve, the vestibular nerve. The vestibular and cochlear nerves travel together from the inner ear to the cerebellopontine angle before entering the brainstem. Here the two nerves separate to synapse in their respective nuclei. The vestibular fibers synapse in the four vestibular nuclei located at the junction of the pons and medulla. From here there are connections to:

- The anterior horn cells of the spinal cord, via the vestibulospinal tract.
- The flocculonodular node of the cerebellum.
- The third, fourth, and sixth ocular motor nuclei, via the medial longitudinal fasciculus.
- The pontine reticular formation.
- The temporal cortex.

Differential diagnosis of dizziness and vertigo

Vertigo is the illusion of movement of either the environment or oneself. The movement may be described as to-and-fro or up-and-down. Often there is accompanying nausea and vomiting. The patient may veer to one side when walking; the gait is more unsteady in the dark or with the eyes closed. Nystagmus is the clinical sign that usually accompanies vertigo. Vertigo may arise from a lesion of the labyrinth, vestibular nerve, cerebellopontine angle, brainstem, cerebellum, or rarely the supranuclear connections (Fig. 9.1).

Labyrinthine failure
Features of labyrinthine failure are as follows:
- Vertigo—occurs in attacks of 1–2 hours duration. There may be accompanying nausea and vomiting.
- Nystagmus—horizontal and/or rotary nystagmus with the fast phase opposite to the side of the lesion.
- Gait—on walking, the patient may veer towards the side of the lesion.
- Hearing—there may be conductive or sensorineural deafness and tinnitus if the auditory pathway is involved.
- Neurologic signs—none.

Ménière's disease
Ménière's disease is characterized by recurrent attacks of vertigo and variable deafness and tinnitus. It occurs in middle age, and, apart from nystagmus and gait disorder, the vertigo is usually self-limiting. It is thought to arise from dilatation of the

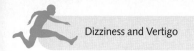
Lesion localization in a patient who presents with vertigo					
	Labyrinthine failure	Vestibular nerve lesion	Cerebellopontine angle lesion	Brainstem lesions	Cerebellar lesions
Vertigo	common short attacks	may be prolonged	rare	may be prolonged	brainstem connections involved
Nystagmus **Fast phase**	horizontal and/or rotary opposite to lesion	horizontal and/or rotary opposite to lesion	horizontal towards lesion	vertical	horizontal towards lesion
Gait	veers towards lesion	veers towards lesion	ataxia towards lesion; hemiparetic	hemiparetic	ataxia towards lesion
Hearing	conductive or sensorineural loss	sensorineural loss	sensorineural high-frequency loss early	unaffected	unaffected
Other neurological signs	none	+/−7th, 5th nerve lesions	5th, 7th, 9th, 10th nerve lesions ipsilateral cerebellar signs contralateral "pyramidal" signs	ipsilateral cranial nerve palsies contralateral "pyramidal" weakness	unilateral cerebellar signs from on ipsilateral cerebellar hemisphere lesion

Fig. 9.1 Differential diagnosis of vertigo and dizziness.

endolymphatic system and degeneration of the organ of Corti. Permanent deafness may occur after repeated attacks.

Benign positional vertigo

Benign positional vertigo arises from dislocation of the otoliths within the posterior semicircular canals. Sudden paroxysms of vertigo occur with movements of the head, particularly lying down, rolling over in bed, bending forward, straightening up, and extending the neck. The vertigo lasts less than a minute and is fatiguable with recurrent movements. The accompanying nystagmus is torsional and similarly fatiguable. Symptoms may be present for several days or months at a time. Some cases seem to follow head trauma or a viral infection of the labyrinth. The Hallpike maneuver can make the diagnosis, and a similar maneuver can sometimes be therapeutic (Fig. 9.2).

Other causes

Other causes of labyrinthine dysfunction include purulent labyrinthitis following meningitis, motion sickness, and toxic effects from alcohol, quinine, and aminoglycosides.

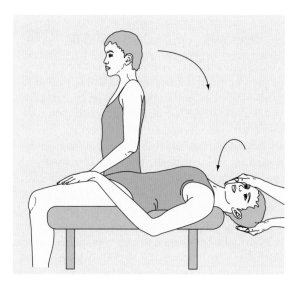

Fig. 9.2 Technique for exhibiting positional nystagmus (Hallpike maneuver).

Vestibular nerve lesions

Features of vestibular nerve lesions are as follows:
- Vertigo—may be severe in vestibular neuronitis (see below).

- Nystagmus—horizontal and/or rotary nystagmus with the fast phase opposite to the side of the lesion.
- Gait—the patient may veer toward the side of the lesion.
- Hearing—sensorineural deafness and tinnitus may occur with involvement of the cochlear nerve.
- Neurologic signs—depending on the etiology, adjacent cranial nerves (e.g., fifth and seventh) may be involved.

The vestibular nerve may be damaged in the petrous temporal bone or the cerebellopontine angle. The latter is dealt with below. Trauma or infection of the petrous temporal bone may involve the seventh and fifth cranial nerves, as may occur with a herpes zoster infection of the nerve or ganglion. Purely vestibular dysfunction occurs in vestibular neuronitis.

Vestibular neuronitis

Vestibular neuronitis manifests as a single severe paroxysm of vertigo without deafness and tinnitus, usually in young or middle-aged adults. Symptoms usually subside within several days but may persist for weeks. An inflammatory etiology is presumptive rather than proven, but the condition frequently follows an upper respiratory tract infection; thus a viral cause has been postulated.

Cerebellopontine angle lesions

Features of cerebellopontine angle lesions are as follows:

- Vertigo—rarely occurs in the early stages.
- Nystagmus—horizontal, coarse, and toward the side of the lesion.
- Gait—ataxic toward the side of the lesion.
- Hearing—high-frequency deafness is often one of the first symptoms.
- Neurologic signs—fifth, seventh, ninth, and tenth nerve palsies, ipsilateral cerebellar signs, and contralateral "pyramidal" weakness.

Causes to consider are acoustic neuroma, other tumors, granulomatous disease, and vascular lesions.

Brainstem lesions

Features of brainstem lesions are as follows:

- Vertigo—may be severe and prolonged.
- Nystagmus—often vertical or multidirectional nystagmus.

- Hearing—usually unaffected since the cochlear and vestibular fibers separate before entering the brainstem.
- Neurologic signs—ipsilateral cranial nerve palsies, contralateral "pyramidal" weakness, and often "cerebellar" ataxia.

Causes include infarction, demyelination, and neoplastic infiltration.

Episodes of vertigo may arise from transient vertebrobasilar ischemia, but it is very rarely the only manifestation of brainstem transient ischemic attacks. Vertigo prior to a typical headache may be part of migraine with aura.

Cerebellar lesions

Features of cerebellar lesions are as follows:

- Vertigo—particularly if the lesion is acute and involving brainstem vestibular connections to the flocculonodular node.
- Nystagmus—horizontal, coarse, and mainly toward the side of the lesion.
- Gait—ataxia of gait with unsteadiness toward the side of the lesion.
- Hearing—unaffected.
- Neurologic signs—unilateral cerebellar signs from an ipsilateral hemisphere lesion.

Causes of cerebellar dysfunction are considered in Chapter 11.

The supranuclear connections

Vertigo may occur as part of the aura of temporal lobe seizures. Uncommonly, it arises from the neck or from ocular motor disorders (ophthalmoplegia).

Other types of dizziness

Vertigo, as described above, is relatively easily recognized. The word dizziness may be used to describe a wide range of other symptoms—light-headedness, a feeling of being on a ship, faintness. Other causes must be considered in the history and examination, including:

- Anxiety with hyperventilation.
- Anemia.
- Hypertension.
- Hypotension—postural (elderly, part of an autonomic neuropathy); cardiac (low-output cardiac failure, arrhythmias).
- Iatrogenic—with or without hypotension.

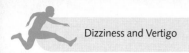
Investigations

The Hallpike maneuver

The Hallpike maneuver is performed with the patient sitting on a bed. The patient's head is positioned 30° to the affected side and taken to 30° below bed level. After a latent period of a few seconds, vertigo is experienced. There is accompanying torsional nystagmus with upper-pole beating towards the floor; the direction of vertigo and nystagmus are reversed on sitting up again. With peripheral (labyrinthine) lesions, symptoms and signs last for about 30 seconds and fatigue with repetition such that they cannot then be reproduced (see Fig. 9.2).

The caloric test

The caloric test is a test of vestibular function. With the patient lying supine, his or her head is raised 30° from horizontal so that the horizontal canals are vertical. Each external meatus is irrigated for 30 seconds with water, first at 30°C, and then, about 5 minutes later, at 44°C. The normal response is **COWS** (after about 20 seconds)—**C**old water results in nystagmus, with the fast phase **O**pposite to the side irrigated; **W**arm water results in nystagmus, with the fast phase to the **S**ame side irrigated.

Two pieces of information can be obtained from the caloric test:

- Canal paresis—no response to irrigation of the external meatus; this occurs in peripheral lesions (i.e., the labyrinth or vestibular ganglion or nerve).
- Directional preponderance—cold water in the left ear and warm in the right will both result in nystagmus to the right. If this response is greater than left-sided nystagmus produced by cold water in the right ear and warm in the left, a right directional preponderance exists. This usually implies a lesion of the brainstem vestibular nuclei on the left.

Bear the following in mind when assessing a patient with vertigo:

- Vertigo is either peripheral or central.
- Vertigo from a supranuclear lesion is uncommon; therefore, the main differential is between a peripheral (labyrinth, vestibular ganglion/nerve) lesion and a brainstem or cerebellar lesion.
- Vertigo is rarely the sole manifestation of brainstem disease—look for symptoms and signs of additional ipsilateral cranial nerve palsies and contralateral "pyramidal" limb weakness.
- Vertigo from a cerebellar lesion may involve signs of cerebellar dysfunction that are absent in vertigo from a lesion of the peripheral vestibular system.
- Vertigo may be the sole symptom of peripheral vestibular dysfunction; this can be confirmed with formal neuro-otological testing.

10. Dysarthria, Dysphonia, and Dysphagia

Definitions

Dysarthria is a disorder of articulation of speech. There is no difficulty in comprehension or expression of language, as in aphasia.

Dysphonia is a disorder of vocalization.

Dysphagia is difficulty with swallowing.

Dysarthria, dysphonia and dysphagia may result from lesions at all levels from the motor cortex down to the numerous muscles involved in articulation, phonation, and swallowing, respectively. The intervening pathways include the basal ganglia, cerebellum, brainstem, cranial nerves, and the neuromuscular junctions (Fig. 10.1).

Remember that local pathology sometimes accounts for these symptoms (e.g., dysarthria due to absence of dentures, dysphagia due to esophageal stricture, dysphonia due to lesions of the vocal cords).

Knowledge of the motor pathways responsible for articulation, phonation, and swallowing enable localization of the site of the lesion.

Differential diagnosis of dysarthria

Articulation involves the use of the respiratory musculature, larynx, pharynx, palate, tongue, and lips. When a word is heard, signals from the primary auditory cortex are received by Wernicke's area (comprehension of speech). From here the signal is transmitted to Broca's area (expression of speech), and then to the motor area of the precentral gyrus, which controls the speech muscles. The motor pathways for articulation therefore arise from the left (dominant hemisphere in most people) precentral gyrus and descend in the corticobulbar tracts to the nuclei of the seventh (motor fibers to the facial muscles, including those of the lips), tenth (nucleus ambiguus—motor fibers to the pharynx, larynx, and soft palate), and twelfth (motor fibers to

the tongue) cranial nerves; and in the corticospinal tracts to the diaphragm and intercostal muscles. The nuclei of the seventh, tenth, and twelfth cranial nerves receive corticobulbar fibers from both the ipsilateral and contralateral hemispheres. As with all movements, articulation is modulated by extrapyramidal influences exerted by the cerebellum and basal ganglia (see Fig. 10.1).

Dysarthria may be caused by a lesion at any level in the above-described pathway. Clinical features of lesions at each level are described below.

Upper motor neuron lesions

The muscles of articulation are bilaterally innervated; therefore, a unilateral lesion may be asymptomatic. A bilateral lesion is usually required to produce significant dysarthria. This may occur at the same event or at separate times. A lesion may interrupt the corticobulbar tract at the level of the motor cortex, internal capsule, midbrain, or pons. This gives rise to a so-called "pseudobulbar palsy."

The speech is slow, indistinct, and forced, often described as "Donald Duck" speech. On examination, the tongue may appear contracted, with limited protrusion. Look for upper motor neuron signs (spasticity in the limbs, brisk reflexes, extensor plantar responses), in particular a brisk jaw jerk. There may also be emotional lability.

Causes of upper motor neuron lesions include:
- Multiple sclerosis.
- Motor neuron disease.
- Cerebral ischemia (middle cerebral artery occlusion).
- Bilateral subcortical ischemic lesions.

Lower motor neuron lesions

Lower motor neuron lesions result from damage to the motor nuclei of the seventh, tenth, and twelfth cranial nerves, or their peripheral extensions (the corresponding cranial nerves), and give rise to a "bulbar palsy." Speech is slurred and indistinct. Labial and lingual sounds are affected. With bilateral

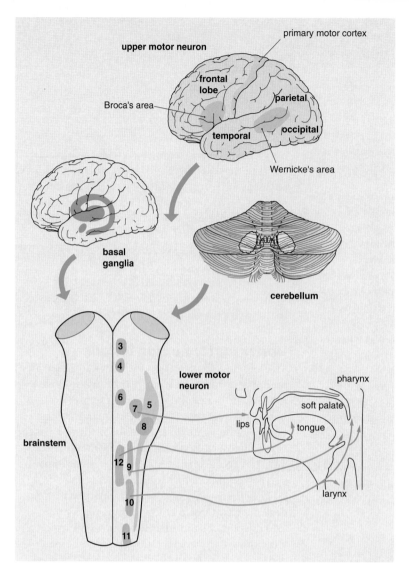

Fig. 10.1 Structures and pathways involved in articulation of speech.

paralysis of the soft palate, the speech gains a nasal quality. The tongue becomes wasted and fasciculates, and the facial muscles are weak.

Causes of lower motor neuron lesions include:
- Guillain Barré syndrome.
- Motor neuron disease.
- Medullary tumors.
- Syringobulbia.
- Poliomyelitis.

Basal ganglia lesions
Akinetic-rigid syndromes
In akinetic-rigid syndromes such as Parkinson's disease, the speech is hypokinetic. It is characterized by rapidly spoken words, which are slurred. The voice is low pitched, monotonous, and without inflection. The speech often trails at the end of sentences.

Chorea and myoclonus
With chorea and myoclonus—as, for example, in Huntington's chorea—the speech is hyperkinetic. It is loud and harsh, intonation is variable, and there is poor coordination of the diaphragm and respiratory muscles, resulting in short breathless sentences.

Athetosis
In patients with athetosis, such as in athetoid cerebral palsy, the speech is loud and slow, and consonants are indistinctly pronounced.

With the above syndromes the diagnosis is often given by the accompanying characteristic movement abnormalities.

Cerebellar lesions

Cerebellar lesions cause ataxic dysarthria. The speech is slow and slurred. This arises from impaired coordination of articulation, which is evident on rapid side-to-side movements of the tongue. Look for other signs of cerebellar dysfunction. If there is also involvement of the corticobulbar tracts, the speech may be "scanning," with words broken up into syllables, which are spoken with varying force.

Causes of cerebellar lesions include:
- Multiple sclerosis.
- Inherited ataxias.
- Alcoholic cerebellar degeneration.

Dysarthria can be caused by a lesion of the:
- Motor cortex (rare).
- Upper motor neuron.
- Basal ganglia.
- Cerebellum.
- Brainstem.
- Lower motor neuron (seventh, tenth and twelth).
- Neuromuscular junction.
- Muscle.
- Oropharynx.

From the features characterizing the dysarthria and additional neurologic signs, it is possible to localize the site of the lesion. Once this has been done, a differential diagnosis of pathologies that can occur at this site can be made. With knowledge of the clinical features of these conditions, history and further examination will narrow the differential diagnosis and prompt the appropriate investigations. It is always wise to inspect the oropharynx first to exclude a local cause for the dysarthria.

Myopathies and disorders of the neuromuscular junction

Both myopathies and disorders of the neuromuscular junction give rise to a dysarthria similar to that of a bulbar palsy.

If there is no evidence of fatiguability (deterioration of the dysarthria at the end of the day, with improvement the following morning), note whether there is a family history of a muscle disorder; look for thinning and weakness of the facial muscles, involvement of the limbs, and for the presence of myotonia. Examples of these disorders are Myasthenia Gravis and myotonic dystrophy.

Oropharyngeal lesions

Local lesions of the oropharynx can cause difficulty with articulation. Examples include:
- Multiple ulcers.
- Oral candidiasis.
- Dental abscess.
- Loose dentures

Differential diagnosis of dysphagia

The descending motor pathway for swallowing closely follows that for articulation.

Dysarthria is therefore often accompanied by dysphagia. Corticobulbar fibers travel to the nuclei of the ninth and tenth cranial nerves. The innervation is again bilateral. Motor fibers from the tenth nucleus supply the soft palate and pharynx, which are required for swallowing; the adjacent ninth nucleus sends motor fibers to the middle constrictor of the pharynx and stylopharyngeus.

A lesion (usually bilateral) interrupting this pathway will cause difficulty with swallowing solids and more so liquids (as opposed to obstruction of the esophagus, which first causes difficulty swallowing solids, and then, as the obstruction progresses, liquids also).

Dysfunction of the swallowing mechanism can be confirmed by videofluoroscopy.

Causes of dysphagia overlap with those for dysarthria, and the two symptoms often coexist, but not invariably so.

Sites of lesions causing dysphagia

Dysphagia can be caused by a lesion of the:
- Bilateral hemisphere (usually vascular).
- Brainstem (multiple sclerosis, vascular, tumors).

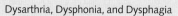
- Cranial nerves (ninth and tenth).
- Neuromuscular junction (myasthenia).
- Muscle (polymyositis).
- Pharynx and esophagus (local pathology).

Differential diagnosis of dysphonia

Phonation is a function of the larynx and the vocal cords. Sound is produced by air passing over the vocal cords; the pitch is altered by changes in tension of the membranous part of the vocal cords, brought about by the intrinsic laryngeal muscles. All are supplied by the laryngeal branches of the tenth cranial nerve (the recurrent laryngeal nerve for all muscles except the cricothyroid, which is supplied by the external laryngeal nerve), which arise from the nucleus ambiguus. The latter has bilateral supranuclear innervation from the corticobulbar fibers. A lesion in this pathway will cause dysphonia (the voice having a husky quality) or aphonia (the inability to produce any sound); with this there is impairment of coughing, which requires normal vocal cord function. Paralysis or a local lesion of the vocal cord can be visualized by indirect laryngoscopy. The paralyzed cord fails to abduct on attempted phonation.

Causes of dysphonia include:
- Medullary lesion involving the nucleus ambiguus—infarction, tumor, syringobulbia.
- Recurrent laryngeal nerve palsy—following thyroid surgery, bronchial carcinoma, aortic aneurysm.
- Vocal cord lesion—polyps, tumor.
- Functional (psychogenic aphonia).

Because of the proximity of the motor pathways governing articulation, swallowing, and phonation, dysfunction of these facilities often accompany one another; for example, a patient with a bulbar palsy may present with dysarthria with nasal intonation, drooling due to difficulty swallowing, and a hoarse voice.

11. Cerebellar Dysfunction

The cerebellum

The cerebellum and its connections are responsible for the coordination of skilled voluntary movement, posture, and gait. The cerebellum can be divided into three functional units (Figs 11.1 and 11.2):

- The flocculonodular lobe (vestibulocerebellum)—phylogenetically the oldest lobe, called the archicerebellum.
- The small anterior lobe, called the paleocerebellum—contains the anterior superior vermis.
- The large posterior lobe, called the neocerebellum—contains the middle part of the vermis.

Peduncles
The fibers entering and leaving the cerebellum form three pairs of cerebellar peduncles. The peduncles attach the cerebellum to the brainstem.

- The inferior cerebellar peduncle (restiform body) contains afferent fibers with one efferent tract—the fastigiobulbar tract to the vestibular nuclei.
- The middle cerebellar peduncle (brachium pontis) contains almost entirely crossed afferents from the contralateral pontine nuclei.
- The superior cerebellar peduncle (brachium conjunctivum) contains efferent fibers.

Connections of the cerebellum
The flocculonodular lobe receives proprioceptive information from the vestibular nuclei; its role is to maintain equilibrium of the body (see Fig. 11.2).

The anterior lobe receives proprioceptive information from the muscles and tendons of the limbs via the dorsal (lower limbs) and ventral (upper limbs) spinocerebellar tracts (the afferent spinocerebellar pathway).

The efferent pathways project to the reticular formation, red nucleus, and vestibular nuclei. The reticulospinal, rubrospinal, and vestibulospinal tracts in turn influence posture, muscle tone, and movement, by regulating activity in the alpha and gamma motor neurons in the spinal cord.

The posterior lobe receives afferent projections from the contralateral cerebral cortex via the pontine nuclei. The efferent pathway is from the Purkinje cells of the cerebellar cortex to the deep intracerebellar nuclei (fastigial, globose, emboliform, and dentate nuclei). From the latter there are projections to the red nucleus and lateral ventral thalamus, and back to the frontal cortex again. Purkinje cells have a purely inhibitory action on the excitatory subcortical intracerebellar nuclei. This pathway allows coordination of skilled movements, which are initiated at the level of the cerebral cortex.

Clinical features of cerebellar dysfunction

Incoordination of movement
Cerebellar dysfunction causes impairment of the process of initiating, stopping, and controlling movements.

This gives rise to ataxia (incoordination) as manifested by the following:

- Intention tremor—there is no tremor at rest, but on intention (e.g., placing the index finger on the nose from rest) there is a coarse oscillating tremor that is more marked as the finger reaches its target.
- Dysdiadochokinesia—inability to carry out rapid alternating movements with regularity.
- Dysmetria—inability to carry out smooth and accurate targeted movements; the latter are jerky, with overshooting of the target, as manifested by the finger—nose and heel—shin tests (see p. 102).

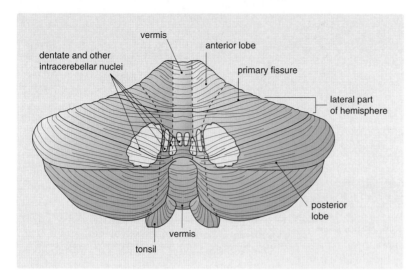

Fig. 11.1 Posterior aspect of the cerebellum.

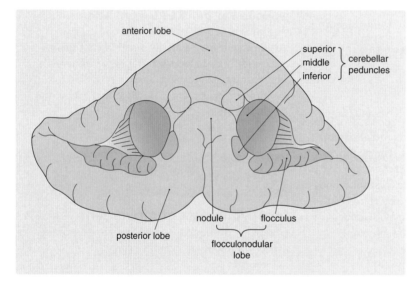

Fig. 11.2 Inferior aspect of the cerebellum, showing the flocculonodular lobe and the three peduncles disconnected from the pons.

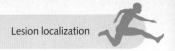

Ataxic gait

The patient walks on a wide base with staggering gait. In mild cases, the unsteadiness may be apparent only when walking heel-to-toe (tandem walking). In a unilateral cerebellar hemisphere lesion, there is unsteadiness towards the side of the lesion. In truncal ataxia there is difficulty sitting or standing without support and the patient tends to fall backwards.

Dysarthric speech

Speech can be slow and slurred or scanning in quality: in scanning speech there is loss of variation of intonation and the words may be broken up into syllables.

Abnormal eye movements

Abnormal eye movements include:
- Jerky pursuits—pursuit movements are slow, with catch-up saccadic movements on attempt to maintain fixation on the moving target.
- Dysmetria of saccades—on attempt to fixate on a target, the eyes overshoot and oscillate several times before fixation is achieved.
- Nystagmus—this is maximal on deviation of the eyes towards the side of the lesion. Nystagmus results from damage of the vestibular connections of the cerebellum.

Titubation

Nodding tremor of the head may occur. This is mainly in the anterior—posterior plane.

Altered posture

A unilateral cerebellar lesion may cause the head (and, when the lesion is recent and severe, the body) to tilt towards the side of the lesion. Head tilt may also be due to a fourth nerve palsy, which can accompany a lesion of the superior medullary vellum (Fig. 11.3).

Hypotonia

Hypotonia is a relatively minor feature of cerebellar diseases, resulting from depression of alpha and gamma motor neuron activity. Hypotonia can sometimes be demonstrated clinically by decreased resistance to passive movement (e.g., extension of a limb), by "pendular" reflexes, or by the rebound phenomenon—with the patient's arms outstretched, his or her forearms are pressed down and then

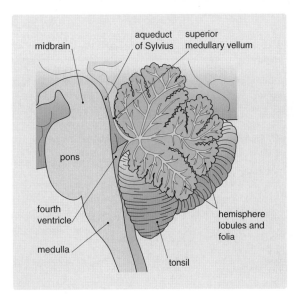

Fig. 11.3 Sagittal section though the cerebellum and brainstem.

abruptly released by the examiner. The arms may rebound upwards much further than usual in the presence of cerebellar hypotonia.

The causes of cerebellar dysfunction and the clinical features resulting from each are listed in Fig. 11.4.

Cerebellar dysfunction is characterized by:
- Ataxia of limb and gait.
- Dysarthria.
- Nystagmus.
- Postural tilt or hypotonia in some patients.

Lesion localization

Cerebellar hemisphere

A lesion of the cerebellar hemisphere causes signs of cerebellar dysfunction in the limbs ipsilateral to the lesion. The gait is ataxic, with a tendency to fall towards the affected side.

Midline structures

Lesions of midline structures cause severe ataxia of gait and stance. Lesion of the vermis causes truncal

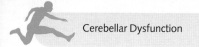

Fig. 11.4 Causes of cerebellar dysfunction.

Causes of cerebellar dysfunction	
Cause	**Additional clinical characteristics**
Tumors	type of tumor—metastatic disease, meningioma, acoustic neuroma, medulloblastoma, hemangioblastoma, paraneoplastic syndrome with bronchial and other carcinomas
Multiple sclerosis	pyramidal, brainstem, and dorsal column signs; optic atrophy
Vascular hemorrhage	history of hypertension, bleeding disorder, on anticoagulants
infarction	history of hypertension, ischemic heart disease, atrial fibrillation, diabetes, hyperlipidemia
Infections abscess	boil or abscess elsewhere, fever, unwell
viral encephalitis	notably varicella within 3 weeks of initial infection
Toxins anti-epileptic drugs	history of epilepsy; signs of acute toxicity or past history of recurrent toxicity
alcohol	acute intoxication; history of chronic abuse, signs of alcoholic liver disease
Metabolic myxedema	myxedematous facies, dry skin and hair, increased weight, cold intolerance, slow-relaxing reflexes, bradycardia
Trauma	head injury
Developmental deformities Arnold-Chiari malformation	pyramidal signs, lower cranial nerve palsies, occipital headache, +/− signs associated with a syrinx
congenital aqueduct stenosis	6th nerve palsies, deafness, papilledema, intellectual decline
Dandy–Walker syndrome	large cystic fourth ventricle resulting in hydrocephalus
Inherited cerebellar ataxias Friedreich's ataxia dominantly inherited ataxias recessively inherited ataxias	pes cavus, pyramidal and dorsal column signs, cardiomyopathy, diabetes, optic atrophy

ataxia, often without the classic triad of limb ataxia, dysarthria, and nystagmus. Lesion of the flocculonodular node causes truncal ataxia, vertigo (vestibular reflex pathways damaged), vomiting (involvement of the floor of the fourth ventricle), and nystagmus, often downbeating.

Space-occupying tumors at midline sites can cause early obstruction of the aqueduct or fourth ventricle. This results in hydrocephalus with headache, vomiting, and papilledema.

12. Tremor and Other Involuntary Movements

Tremor is the most frequently encountered involuntary movement and often arises from a systemic medical cause rather than a focal neurologic disorder.

The nontremulous basal ganglia movement disorders are chorea, athetosis, dystonia, and tics. Myoclonic jerks (myoclonus), like tremor, can be symptomatic of a range of conditions, which include systemic disease as well as specific neurologic disorders. Each of these is discussed below.

Tremor

Tremor is a steady rhythmic oscillatory movement of the muscles. Tremor may be normal (physiologic) or abnormal (pathologic). With a physiologic tremor, all muscle groups are affected, although it is most commonly noted in the hands. The tremor is present during waking and sleeping hours and has a frequency of 8 to 13 Hz. With a pathologic tremor, there may be involvement of the limb extremities, head (including jaw, tongue, lips, and vocal cords), and trunk. The symptoms are present during waking hours only, and the tremor frequency is slower, usually between 4 and 7 Hz.

When assessing a patient with a tremor, the first step is to distinguish whether the tremor occurs at rest, with postural change, or on movement (Fig. 12.1). This can be best assessed by observing any movements at rest and asking the patient to stretch out his or her arms in front of him or her and then, from this position, to place the index fingers on the tip of his or her nose. A postural tremor is accentuated by holding the hands outstretched; a parkinsonian tremor may improve in that position and during action, being usually most noticeable at rest.

Resting tremor
Parkinsonian tremor is a coarse, "pill-rolling" tremor that occurs at rest and often improves with movement. It is usually observed in the hands and arms on one or both sides (see Fig. 23.2, p. 138); the feet and head may also be involved. Other signs of Parkinson's disease should be noted, e.g., shuffling gait, loss of arm swing, immobile facies, rigidity and bradykinesia of the limbs (see Fig. 23.4). There is little correspondence between the latter features and the degree of tremor. The tremor may respond to anticholinergic drugs.

Postural tremor
Physiologic tremor
Physiologic tremor may be exaggerated by :
- Anxiety.
- Metabolic disturbances—hyperthyroidism, pheochromocytoma.
- Alcohol withdrawal.
- Drugs—lithium, sodium valproate, sympathomimetics, tea and coffee.

Beta-blockers may diminish a physiologic tremor.

Essential tremor
Essential tremor may be difficult to distinguish from an exaggerated physiologic tremor. It tends to involve the upper limbs, but the head and trunk may later be involved. It may be familial, inherited in an autosomal dominant manner, in which case it may present in childhood or early adulthood. If there is no family history it is termed essential tremor. If it occurs late in life it is called senile tremor. Notably there is temporary improvement with alcohol.

Therapeutically an essential tremor responds to beta-blockers and sometimes barbiturates or benzodiazepines.

Intention tremor
Cerebellar tremor
Cerebellar dysfunction (see Chapter 11) will give rise to a coarse action tremor. It is absent at rest and appears on movement. On performing the finger—nose test, the finger oscillates with increasing amplitude on approaching the target. Rhythmic

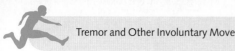

Fig. 12.1 Summary of movement disorders.

Summary of movement disorders		
Tremor rhythmic biphasic oscillatory movements of the muscles	resting	parkinsonian tremor
	postural	physiological, benign essential tremor
	intention	cerebellar, red nucleus tremor
Chorea rapid, irregular, jerky movements **Athetosis** slow, writhing purposeless movements chorea and athetosis often occur together—choreoathetosis		iatrogenic Huntington's chorea Sydenham's chorea Wilson's disease hyperthyroidism polycythemia vera systemic lupus erthromatosis
Dystonia	generalized	dystonia musculorum deformans iatrogenic Wilson's disease paroxysmal dystonia
	focal	spasmodic torticollis blepharospasm oromandibular dystonia writer's cramp
Hemiballismus unilateral violent flinging movements of the proximal limb muscles		tumor infarction
Myoclonus brief shock-like muscular contractions that are usually irregular and asymmetrical		myoclonic epilepsy essential myoclonus progressive myoclonus—lipid storage diseases, Creutzfeldt–Jakob disease, hepatic failure static myoclonus—post-viral, anoxic
Asterixis arrhythmic flexion movements of the dorsiflexed hands with arms outstretched		hepatic encephalopathy uremic encephalopathy hypercapnia
Akathisia restlessness arising from an irresistible desire to move		neuroleptic therapy
Tic repetitive brief contraction of a muscle or group of muscles		

oscillation of the head and trunk (titubation) may occur. Other signs of cerebellar dysfunction should be noted.

Red nucleus tremor

A red nucleus tremor is a coarse and often violent tremor. Slight movement of the arm may precipitate a wide-amplitude tremor of the limb. This type of tremor arises from vascular or demyelinating lesions affecting the dentorubrothalamic tract.

Cerebellar and red nucleus tremors do not respond to anticholinergics or beta-blockers.

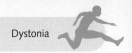

Stereotactic lesions of the contralateral ventrolateral thalamus may abolish pathologic tremors.

Asterixis

Asterixis is the flapping of hands observed with arms outstretched and hands dorsiflexed. The flap occurs several times a minute and is incorrectly termed a tremor ("flapping tremor"). It is seen in metabolic encephalopathies (e.g., hepatic, uremic) and hypercapnia.

Chorea and athetosis

Chorea consists of rapid, irregular, jerky movements affecting the face, trunk, and limbs.

Athetosis refers to slow, writhing movements which affect all muscle groups, particularly those of the face and upper limbs.

The two types of movement disorder often occur together, hence the term choreoathetosis. The disorder arises from disease of the basal ganglia.

Causes of choreoathetosis
Causes of choreoathetosis include:
- Drugs—levodopa, phenothiazines, butyrophenones, oral contraceptives.
- Huntington's chorea.
- Sydenham's chorea.
- Senile chorea.
- Metabolic disorder—Wilson's disease.
- Endocrine disorder—hyperthyroidism.
- Hematologic disorder—polycythemia vera.
- Vascular disorders—systemic lupus erythematosus, infarction.
- Cerebral palsy.

Tardive dyskinesia
Long-term treatment with drugs such as phenothiazines and butyrophenones may result in development of choreoathetoid movements of the face, mouth, tongue, and limbs. Withdrawal of the drug is followed by a period of deterioration before improvement is seen. Unfortunately, despite withdrawal, the symptoms frequently persist.

Dystonia

Dystonia is prolonged muscular contraction on attempted voluntary movement, which results in abnormal posturing. Dystonias may be generalized or focal (see Fig. 12.1). The site of the pathology is the basal ganglia.

Generalized dystonias
Causes of generalized dystonia include:
- Dystonia musculorum deformans—the disorder is familial (autosomal dominant or recessive). The dystonias may initially be focal and intermittent, but eventually there is constant dystonia of the head, trunk, and limbs.
- Drugs—phenothiazines, butyrophenones, levodopa, metoclopramide (focal or generalized).
- Symptomatic dystonia (secondary to other diseases)—Wilson's disease, cerebral palsy following hypoxic damage or kernicterus.
- Paroxysmal dystonia—familial condition of brief attacks of dystonic posturing provoked by sudden noise or movement.

Focal dystonias
Examples of focal dystonias include:
- Cervical dystonia ("spasmodic torticollis")—involuntary movement of the neck toward one side, in extension (retrocollis) or flexion (anterocollis). The contracting muscles may become painful. The sternomastoid and trapezius are most affected and may eventually hypertrophy.
- Blepharospasm—a series of involuntary clonic contractions of the eyelid muscles.
- Oromandibular dystonia—involuntary dystonic movements of the mouth, tongue, or jaw can affect women in the sixth decade of life. It may also occur in patients on long-term neuroleptic therapy, the elderly, and the developmentally delayed.
- Writer's cramp—attempt at writing is prevented by spasm of the muscles of the hand, which may be painful. The symptoms can spread to the forearm and shoulders. On stopping the activity, the spasm resolves. Other focal occupational dystonias occur in musicians and sportsmen, similarly affecting highly skilled movements.

The most effective treatment for focal dystonias is botulinum toxin injections into the affected muscles at 3-month intervals.

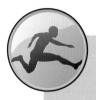 Clinically, it may be difficult to differentiate chorea, athetosis, and dystonia because they often occur together.

Hemiballismus

Hemiballismus describes unilateral sudden violent flinging movements of the proximal limb muscles. It results from a lesion of the contralateral subthalamic nucleus (e.g., infarction, tumor).

Myoclonus

Myoclonic jerks are shock-like, asymmetrical muscular contractions that occur irregularly. There is often particular sensitivity to various stimuli, which may precipitate the jerks (e.g., a sudden noise, light, touch, or voluntary movement). The symptoms settle during sleep.

Causes of myoclonus
Causes of myoclonus include:
- Myoclonic epilepsy.
- Essential myoclonus.

- Progressive myoclonus (myoclonus with a progressive encephalopathy): familial metabolic disorders—lipid-storage diseases (sialidosis, Gaucher's disease); degenerative disease—Creutzfeldt–Jakob disease, subacute sclerosing panencephalitis; metabolic disorder—hepatic and uremic encephalopathies.
- Static myoclonus—anoxic, postviral.
- Medications—gabapentin.

Habit spasms and tics

A tic is the repetitive brief contraction of a muscle or group of muscles. Multiple tics constitute one of the most notable tic syndromes, Gilles de la Tourette syndrome. This is characterized by involuntary snorting, grunting, verbal obscenities, and aggressive and sexual impulses. It responds to haloperidol.

Habit spasms are habitual movements that a person feels the need to make to relieve tension and may be suppressed voluntarily (e.g., sniffing, blinking).

Akathisia

Akathisia is characterized by an irresistible desire to move, with consequent restlessness. It is seen in patients on neuroleptic drugs. Neurologic examination is usually normal.

13. Limb Weakness

Weakness in the limbs can result from pathology anywhere along the upper motor neuron (UMN) pathway (motor cortex, subcortical fibers, brainstem, or spinal cord), from a lesion of the lower motor neuron (LMN; anterior horn cell, nerve root, plexus, or peripheral nerve), or from disorders of the neuromuscular junctions or the muscles themselves. The distribution of weakness and other distinctive physical signs usually allow differentiation of these various levels of involvement. Many patients use the word weakness to describe other deficits that are not actually characterized by a lack of power, such as parkinsonism, ataxia, fatigue, and clumsiness due to sensory loss. Here again, a skilled examination is an essential complement to the clinical history.

Terminology

Paralysis is the partial or complete loss of voluntary movement. Related terms are plegia, palsy, and paresis, although the latter is most appropriate to describe incomplete paralysis, the most common type of weakness in practice.

- Monoparesis is weakness of the muscles of one arm or leg.
- Hemiparesis is weakness of the muscles of the arm and leg on one side of the body, often with facial weakness on the affected side.
- Paraparesis is weakness of both legs.
- Tetraparesis is weakness of both arms and legs

Upper motor neuron weakness

UMN weakness results from damage of the corticospinal tract at any point from the motor cortex to the spinal cord (Fig. 13.1). If the lesion occurs above the decussation of the fibers at the level of the medullary pyramids, the weakness will be contralateral to the site of the lesion. If it occurs below this level, the signs will be ipsilateral.

The following clinical features characterize a UMN lesion.

Increased tone

Initially, the paralysis may be flaccid (with absent or diminished tendon reflexes). Increased tone (spasticity) develops after hours, days, or, very rarely, weeks. This is manifested by:

- "Catch"—mild spasticity may be detected as a "catch" in the pronators on passive supination of the forearm and in the flexors of the hand on extension of the wrist.
- The "clasp-knife" phenomenon—following strong resistance to passive flexion of the knee, there is sudden relaxation of the extensor muscles of the lower limbs.
- Clonus—rhythmic involuntary muscular contractions follow an abruptly applied and sustained stretch stimulus, e.g., at the ankle following sudden passive dorsiflexion of the foot.

"Pyramidal-pattern" weakness

The antigravity muscles are predominantly affected, i.e., the flexors of the upper limbs and the extensors of the lower limbs; thus the characteristic posture of the arms flexed and pronated, and the legs extended and adducted (Fig. 13.2).

Absence of muscle wasting and fasciculations

Muscle wasting and fasciculations are features of a LMN lesion.

Brisk tendon reflexes and extensor plantar responses

The tendon reflexes are brisk. The cremasteric and abdominal reflexes are depressed or absent. The plantar responses are extensor (upgoing toes).

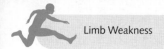
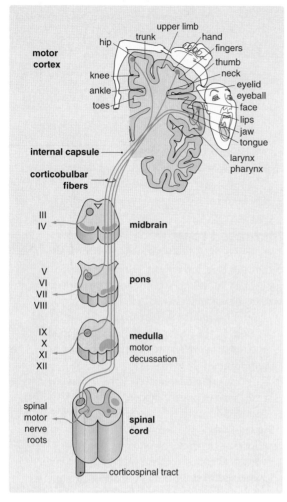

Fig. 13.1 Descending motor pathways from the cortex to the brainstem, cranial nerves, and spinal cord.

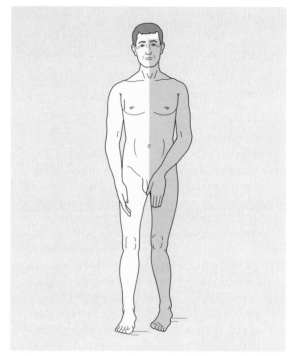

Fig. 13.2 "Pyramidal" pattern of weakness causing a characteristic posture of the left arm (partially flexed) and leg (extended) after a right hemisphere stroke.

Patterns of upper motor neuron weakness

Hemiparesis

Hemiparesis results from unilateral lesions of the contralateral cerebral hemisphere or brainstem (when the face is usually also affected) or from an ipsilateral lesion in the lower medulla or high cervical cord (when the face is spared) (Fig. 13.3).

Associated clinical features such as dysphasia, sensory disturbance, or cranial nerve involvement will usually distinguish hemisphere and brainstem lesions from those in the spinal cord (see Fig. 13.3). By far the most common cause of hemiparesis is a stroke involving the cerebral hemisphere, whether it be the cortex or internal capsule (see Fig. 13.3).

Tetraparesis

Spastic (UMN) weakness of all four limbs results from lesions in the brainstem (infarction, multiple sclerosis, tumor) or cervical cord (spondylosis, prolapsed intervertebral disc, multiple sclerosis, tumor). Brainstem pathology will be recognized from additional weakness of the cranial muscles (ocular, facial, or bulbar, depending on the level of the lesion), often with other corresponding brainstem cranial nerve symptoms such as diplopia, facial numbness, vertigo, dysarthria and dysphagia.

Spastic tetraparesis results most often from cervical spondylosis, multiple sclerosis, and traumatic cord lesions; less often from other pathologies such as tumors, arteriovenous malformations (AVMs), or rheumatoid disease at the atlantoaxial (C1/C2) junction. In cervical spondylotic myelopathy, there are often additional LMN signs in the arms, resulting from compression of nerve roots within their exit foramina, most often at C5–C7 levels.

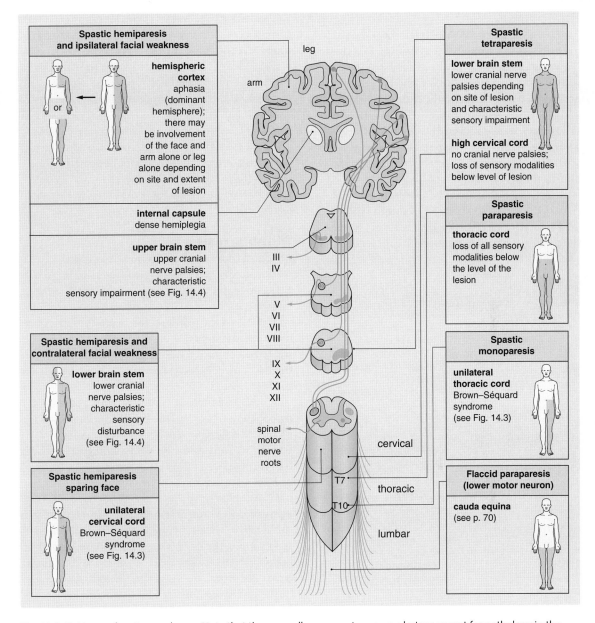

Fig. 13.3 Patterns of motor weakness. Note that these are all upper motor neuron lesions except for pathology in the cauda equina, which damages multiple lumbar and sacral nerve roots.

Weakness of all four limbs may also result from:
- Generalized LMN disorders (generalized anterior horn cell involvement such as in polio, generalized peripheral nerve involvement as in a motor neuropathy).
- Disorders of the neuromuscular junction (Myasthenia Gravis).
- Muscle disease (polymyositis).

The term flaccid tetraparesis would then sometimes be applied.

Tetraparesis in motor neuron disease is usually due to a combination of UMN (corticospinal pathway) and LMN (anterior horn cell) involvement (see pp. 70–74 for further discussion of LMN lesions; also see Fig. 13.7.)

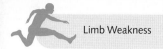

Paraparesis

Paraparesis is usually a UMN syndrome—spastic paraparesis—due to spinal cord disease. Even lesions in the cervical region will often cause spasticity, mainly in the legs, sometimes with LMN signs in the arms, which correspond to the segmental level of the pathology (spondolysis, prolapsed intervertebral disc, tumor, motor neuron disease). Spastic paraparesis is often encountered in clinical exams as well as real life, and a systematic approach to the numerous causes is important (Fig. 13.4).

A rare cause of bilateral UMN symptoms and signs in the legs, resembling a spinal cord syndrome, is a cerebral lesion involving both cortical leg areas in the parasagittal region of the brain. This is classically a meningioma, but sagittal sinus thrombosis and the form of cerebral palsy known as congenital spastic diplegia are other examples.

Flaccid (LMN) paraparesis results from lesions in the cauda equina (central disc prolapse, tumor). The diagnosis is usually clear from the accompanying severe sphincter dysfunction and sensory impairment over sacral and lower lumbar dermatomes (see Fig. 13.3 and p. 162). If the tip of the spinal cord (conus) is involved as well, there may also be some UMN signs in the form of brisk knee jerks and extensor plantar responses, but with flaccid tone and absent ankle jerks.

Monoparesis

Localized cerebral cortical lesions may cause weakness confined to one contralateral limb, typically the leg and foot with a parasagittal tumor or infarct.

A stroke in the middle cerebral artery territory is much more common and will sometimes cause weakness confined to the upper limb, but usually there is some UMN facial weakness as well, even if the leg is spared.

A unilateral thoracic cord lesion may present with monoparesis of the leg (see Fig. 13.3). There will usually be reflex and sensory findings of a Brown–Séquard syndrome to clarify the diagnosis (see Fig. 14.3).

Monoparesis is much more commonly due to LMN pathology involving the anterior horn cells (early motor neuron disease), cervical or lumbar spinal nerve roots (prolapsed intervertebral disc, spondylosis), the brachial or lumbar plexus, or peripheral nerves. The weakness in these conditions is therefore focal, involving specific muscles within the limb, and accompanied by wasting and often fasciculation, and loss of the appropriate tendon reflex(es) (see Fig. 13.7).

Causes of spastic paraparesis	
spinal cord compression	cervical spondylosis cervical or thoracic disc metastatic tumor primary tumor (meningioma, neurofibroma) infective (epidural abscess, spinal TB) epidural hematoma
inflammatory disorders	multiple sclerosis idiopathic transverse myelitis sarcoidosis infections (Lyme, zoster, TB, AIDS)
degenerative disorders	motor neuron disease syringomyelia
vascular	spinal cord infarction vasculitis, systemic lupus erythematosus spinal AVM
trauma	cord contusion, laceration or transection displaced vertebral fracture or disc traumatic epidural hematoma
metabolic/nutritional	B_{12} deficiency (subacute combined degeneration)
rare hereditary conditions	Friedreich's ataxia hereditary spastic paraparesis
parasagittal brain lesions	meningioma cerebral venous sinus thrombosis congenital spastic diplegia

Fig. 13.4 Causes of spastic paraparesis.

Lower motor neuron weakness

LMN damage can occur at the level of the anterior horn cells, their axons in the anterior nerve roots, the plexi, or the peripheral nerves. LMN weakness is characterized by the following features.

Decreased tone
Tone is typically reduced, particularly when muscle wasting has occurred.

Focal pattern of weakness and wasting

LMN weakness can occur in individual muscles as well as groups of muscles. The denervated muscle becomes atrophied, and wasting is evident within 2 to 3 weeks of onset. The pattern of weakness and wasting depends on the site of the lesion:

- Anterior horn cell disease eventually causes generalized weakness and wasting; however, it can begin distally in either an arm or leg such that it mimics a peripheral nerve lesion (e.g., an ulnar nerve palsy).
- Nerve root lesions result in weakness in the respective myotomes and wasting in a segmental distribution corresponding to the root involved.
- A plexus lesion causes weakness and wasting in the distribution of more than one nerve root, i.e., corresponding to the roots involved in the damaged part of the plexus.
- In a peripheral nerve lesion, weakness and wasting will be restricted to the muscles innervated by the nerve.

Fasciculations

Fasciculations are brief contractions of motor units that can be seen through the skin. They are present in weak and wasted muscles; they are particularly prevalent in motor neuron disease.

Pain and sensory disturbance

Sensory changes often occur in lesions of the nerve root, plexus, and peripheral nerve. In such situations, nerve root and plexus lesions are often accompanied by pain. There are no sensory signs in motor neuron disease.

Reduced tendon reflexes and flexor plantar responses

Tendon reflexes are reduced or lost depending on the distribution of LMN involvement. Abdominal and cremasteric reflexes are unaffected. Plantar responses are flexor.

Patterns of lower motor neuron weakness

Motor neuron (anterior horn cell) disease

Weakness caused by anterior horn cell disease may be diffuse or confined to a restricted group of muscles. An important feature to observe is the prominent fasciculations. Anterior horn cell disease may be:

- Genetic (e.g., spinal muscular atrophy).
- Idiopathic (e.g., amyotrophic lateral sclerosis, motor neuron disease). Note that if there is also involvement of the corticobulbar and corticospinal fibers, UMN signs will also be present.
- Infective (e.g., poliomyelitis).
- Toxic.

Radiculopathy (root lesions) and plexopathy (plexus lesions)

To differentiate the site of a root or plexus lesion requires knowledge of the myotomes (see Fig. 17.11 and Fig. 17.12).

A root lesion will cause muscle weakness in the corresponding myotome). If the dorsal root is also involved, there will be accompanying segmental sensory loss in the defined dermatome (see Fig. 14.2).

A plexus lesion will cause weakness in muscles innervated by a number of nerve roots which comprise the plexus. There may be accompanying sensory loss over several dermatomes corresponding to the affected nerve roots (see Fig. 13.7)

Examples of plexus lesions
Brachial plexus
Lesions of the brachial plexus (Fig. 13.5) include:

- Erb's palsy (C5, C6)—upper plexus injury (loss of shoulder abduction and elbow flexion).

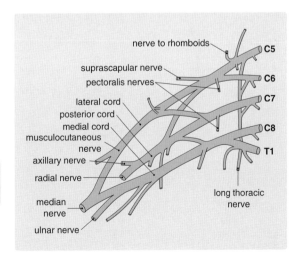

Fig. 13.5 The brachial plexus.

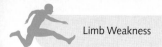
- Klumpke's palsy (C8, T1)—lower plexus injury (loss of function of the intrinsic muscles of the hand and long flexors and extensors of the fingers).

Both Erb's and Klumpke's palsy can arise from traction of the arm at birth.

Other lesions of the brachial plexus include:

- Thoracic outlet syndrome—the brachial plexus and the subclavian artery and vein are compressed by a fibrous band or cervical rib.
- Neuralgic amyotrophy—an acute brachial plexus neuropathy which may follow infection, inoculation, or surgery. The weakness and wasting in the arm is usually preceded by severe pain.

Lumbosacral plexus

Lesions of the lumbosacral plexus (Fig.13.6) include:

- Trauma following abdominal or pelvic surgery.
- Infiltration by neoplasia or granulomatous disease.
- Compression from an abdominal aortic aneurysm.

Disorders of the peripheral nerves

Disorders of the peripheral nerves include:

- Mononeuropathy—disease of a single peripheral nerve (e.g., lesion of the median nerve from compression in the carpal tunnel, lesion of the common peroneal nerve from trauma involving the fibular head).
- Multifocal neuropathy—this is the term used when many single nerves are involved, such as occurs in diabetes, sarcoid, leprosy, vasculitic disease, and neoplasia.
- Polyneuropathy (also termed peripheral neuropathy)—this is the more widespread involvement of the peripheral nerves, typically in a symmetrical distal distribution (e.g., diabetic neuropathy, Guillain Barré syndrome, vitamin B_{12} deficiency, drugs such as isoniazid).

Patterns of weakness caused by these disorders are shown in Fig. 13.7.

Disorders of the neuromuscular junction

These include Myasthenia Gravis, Eaton–Lambert syndrome, and iatrogenic syndromes; the latter two are rare.

The weakness predominantly affects the proximal muscles of the limb girdle, but it becomes more widespread in advanced disease. In Myasthenia Gravis, the ocular muscles are primarily affected; there may be weakness of the proximal limb, and the bulbar and respiratory muscles.

The characteristic feature is fatiguability of muscle strength, which is clinically demonstrable. Wasting is uncommon, occurring in 15% of cases. Reflexes are seldom affected; plantar responses are flexor (Fig. 13.8).

Myopathy (disorders of the muscle)

In a myopathy, the limb weakness is bilateral and proximal in the upper and/or lower limbs. (The main exception is myotonic dystrophy, where characteristically the distal limb muscles are affected.) The face, neck, and trunk are often involved.

Muscle pain and cramps can occur after exercise in some myopathies.

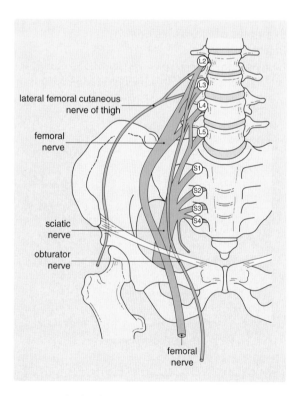

Fig. 13.6 The lumbosacral plexus.

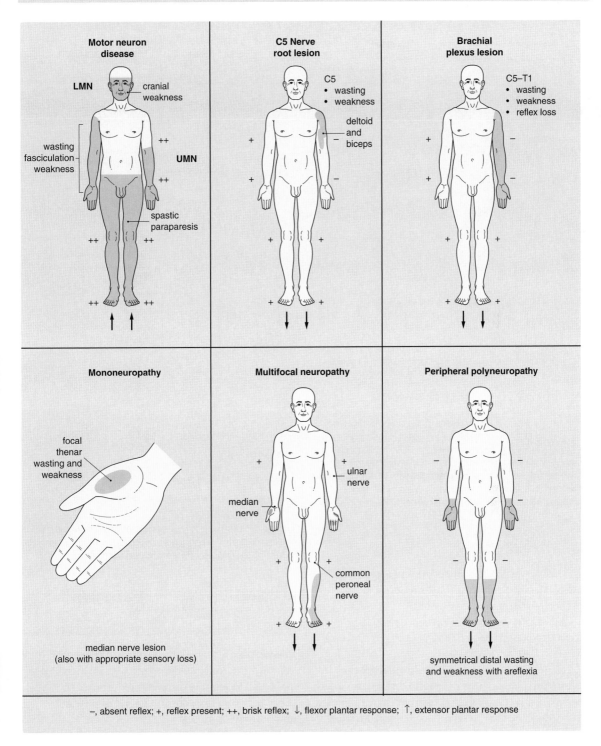

Fig. 13.7 Patterns of weakness due to lower motor neuron lesions.

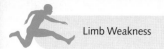

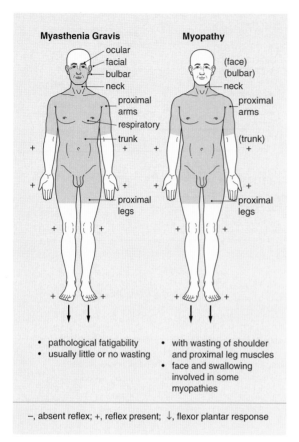

Myasthenia Gravis

ocular
facial
bulbar
neck
proximal arms
respiratory
trunk

- pathological fatigability
- usually little or no wasting

Myopathy

(face)
(bulbar)
neck
proximal arms
(trunk)
proximal legs

- with wasting of shoulder and proximal leg muscles
- face and swallowing involved in some myopathies

−, absent reflex; +, reflex present; ↓, flexor plantar response

Fig. 13.8 Pattern of weakness in neuromuscular junction diseases (Myasthenia) and in myopathies. In both cases, the tendon reflexes are preserved unless weakness is severe, and sensation is, of course, intact.

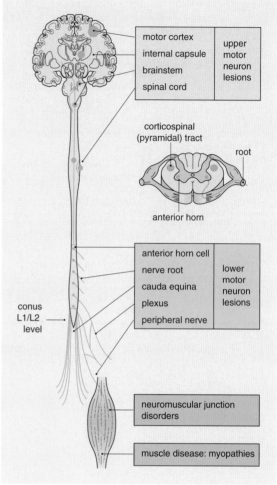

motor cortex	upper motor neuron lesions
internal capsule	
brainstem	
spinal cord	

corticospinal (pyramidal) tract

root

anterior horn

conus L1/L2 level

anterior horn cell	lower motor neuron lesions
nerve root	
cauda equina	
plexus	
peripheral nerve	

neuromuscular junction disorders

muscle disease: myopathies

Fig. 13.9 Summary of lesions causing muscle weakness via the upper motor neuron corticospinal (pyramidal) tract, the lower motor neuron, or neuromuscular structures.

Muscle wasting may be severe and is restricted to the weak muscle groups. Tone is reduced in proportion to the muscle wasting.

Reflexes are reduced in advanced muscle weakness but unaffected in the early stages; plantar responses are flexor.

There are no sensory signs in disorders of the neuromuscular junction or muscle. In the later stages of a myopathy (and rarely in neuromuscular junction disorders), the clinical signs may be similar to that of an LMN lesion. The differentiation can be made from the distribution of the muscle weakness and features of the history (see Fig. 13.8).

Overview of conditions causing limb weakness

The possible levels of involvement of the motor system are summarized in Fig. 13.9, in which UMN and LMN lesions are distinguished from each other and from disorders of the neuromuscular junction and of muscle.

Patients with fatigue may complain of weakness. However, on formal examination these patients have full power and neurologic examination is normal.

14. Limb Sensory Symptoms

As in the case of weakness, sensory symptoms can arise from lesions at various levels within the central nervous system (cortex, subcortex, thalamus, brainstem, spinal cord) or from lesions of the peripheral sensory pathway (nerve root, plexus, peripheral nerve). The anatomical distribution of sensory disturbance, sometimes its quality and timing, and the finding of other physical signs will usually enable a topographic diagnosis to be made. Knowledge of the anatomy of the main sensory pathways is an essential prerequisite for this diagnostic process (Fig. 14.1).

Fibers that carry sensory information travel in cutaneous sensory or sensorimotor nerves. The nerve endings contain different receptors adapted to respond to a variety of sensory stimuli. There are two main pathways for the appreciation of different modalities of sensation:

- The dorsal (posterior) column pathway.
- The spinothalamic pathway.

The dorsal (posterior) column pathway

The dorsal column pathway carries information concerned with light touch, two-point discrimination, vibration, and proprioception. Fibers carrying this information travel from the cutaneous nerves to the dorsal ganglia, where the cell bodies lie. Fibers from the dorsal ganglia enter the spinal cord via the dorsal nerve roots, and synapse in the dorsal horn. From here they ascend in the dorsal columns and terminate in the gracile and cuneate nuclei of the medulla. The fibers decussate in the medulla and travel upward to synapse in the thalamus and thence the parietal cortex. A somatotopic order is maintained throughout the pathway from the spinal cord to parietal cortex.

With lesions of this pathway, the patient may complain of numbness, "pins and needles", a burning sensation, or incoordination of the hands or gait due to loss of proprioceptive information.

The spinothalamic pathway

The spinothalamic pathway carries information about pain and temperature. Itch and tickle are also carried by this pathway. The fibers travel with those concerned with other sensory modalities, within the peripheral nerves to the dorsal root ganglia and dorsal nerve roots (see Fig. 14.1). The fibers ascend or descend for one or two segments in Lissauer's tract before synapsing in the dorsal horn. At this level they decussate and ascend in the opposite spinothalamic tract, to synapse in the thalamus and ultimately the parietal cortex. Again, a somatotopic order is maintained throughout the central pathway.

Clinical manifestations of lesions of this pathway may include paraesthesia, pain, or the acquisition of injuries due to impaired pain perception, e.g., burns and excessive wearing of the joints (which become deformed as a result—Charcot's joints), and trophic changes such as cold hands and feet with brittle, damaged nails.

Sensory syndromes

Sensory symptoms may arise from a lesion involving the peripheral nerves, the dorsal nerve roots, dorsal ganglia, or the central pathways. Lesions of the central pathways can be considered at the level of the spinal cord, brainstem, thalamus, and parietal cortex.

Lesions of peripheral nerves
Mononeuropathy
In a mononeuropathy, damage to a sensory nerve is accompanied by sensory impairment of all modalities in the corresponding anatomical distribution (Fig.

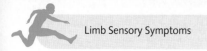

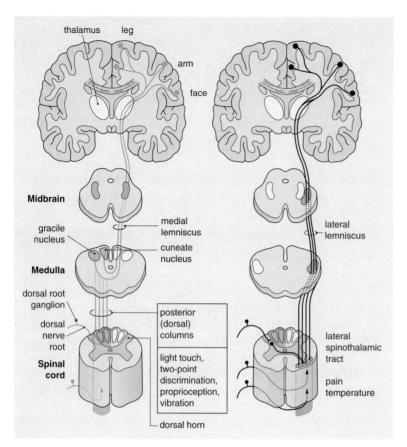

Fig. 14.1 Anatomy of the main sensory pathways in the spinal cord. Note that dorsal column fibers ascend on the ipsilateral side of the spinal cord and decussate in the medulla, whereas spinothalamic fibers cross the central gray matter of the spinal cord (after synapsing in the dorsal horn) and ascend on the opposite side of the cord.

14.2). If a mixed motor and sensory nerve is involved, there will also be weakness of the muscles supplied by the nerve (see Chapter 28).

Multifocal neuropathy

Multifocal neuropathy may involve a number of individual nerves and occurs, for example, in diabetes, sarcoidosis, vasculitis, leprosy, amyloidosis, and carcinomatous disease.

Polyneuropathy

In a polyneuropathy, symmetrical sensory impairment of all modalities occurs in a distal pattern involving the hands, feet, and legs, characteristically termed a "glove-and-stocking" sensory loss. The reflexes are diminished or lost and there may be accompanying muscle weakness. Causes of a polyneuropathy include diabetes, chronic alcohol abuse, vitamin B_{12} deficiency, amyloidosis, and drugs (isoniazid, heavy metals, antineoplastic agents).

Lesions of the dorsal nerve roots and ganglia

Each dorsal nerve root carries sensory fibers of all modalities from a segmental area, a dermatome, on that side of the body (Fig. 14.2). Since there is overlap from adjacent roots, lesions of a single nerve root will not result in complete loss of sensation within the defined dermatome; this requires involvement of two or more adjacent roots. The corresponding tendon reflexes may be diminished or lost. Muscle weakness of lower motor neuron type occurs if the anterior roots are also involved; this is more common in plexus lesions.

Examples include reactivation of the herpes zoster virus (shingles) and a prolapsed intervertebral disc.

Lesions of the spinal cord

Sensory disturbances arising from lesions of the spinal cord are illustrated in Fig. 14.3.

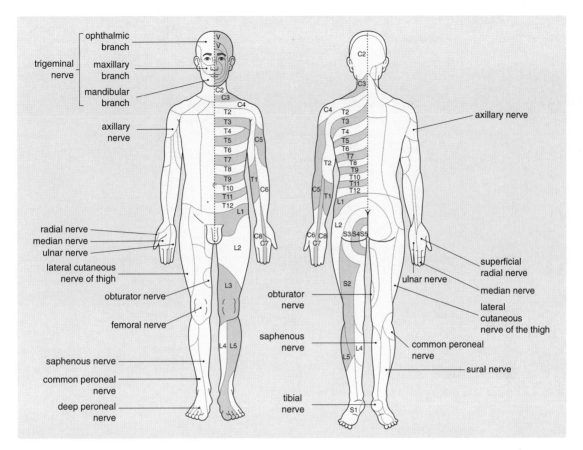

Fig. 14.2 Distribution of sensory dermatomes and the territories of individual peripheral nerves that may be affected by mononeuropathy.

Transection of the cord

Transection of the cord causes bilateral impairment of all sensory modalities below the level of transection (as defined by the dermatomal pattern in Fig. 14.2); pain and temperature loss may begin one or two segments below this level. There is initially a flaccid, and eventually a spastic, paraplegia or tetraplegia (depending on the level of transection).

Lesion of the posterior spinal cord

A lesion of the posterior spinal cord affects the dorsal columns, with sparing of the spinothalamic and corticospinal fibers. There is impaired light touch, two-point discrimination, vibration, and proprioception below the level of the lesion. Motor function, and perception of pain and temperature are spared unless the lesion progresses to involve the anterior part of the cord. Examples include compression by a prolapsed intervertebral disc.

Lesion of the anterior cord

A lesion of the anterior cord affects the spinothalamic and corticospinal tracts, with sparing of the dorsal columns. There is bilateral impairment of pain and temperature perception and a spastic paraplegia or tetraplegia below the level of the lesion. Examples include occlusion of the anterior spinal artery (artery of Adamkiewicz with aortic dissection).

Hemisection of the cord (Brown–Séquard syndrome)

Hemisection of the cord causes impairment of light touch, two-point discrimination, vibration, and proprioception below the level of the lesion on the same side; and impaired perception of pain and temperature on the opposite side. Involvement of one or more nerve roots at the site of the lesion will result in impairment of all sensory modalities on that

77

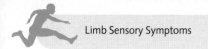

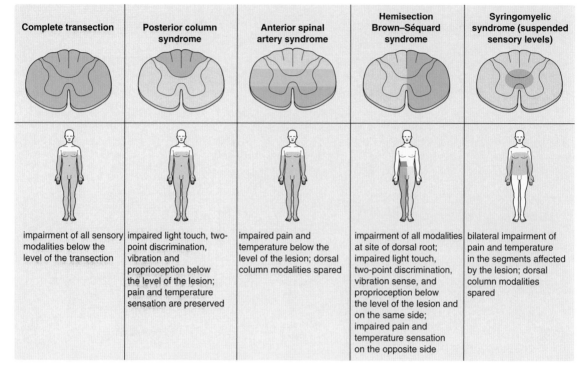

Complete transection	Posterior column syndrome	Anterior spinal artery syndrome	Hemisection Brown–Séquard syndrome	Syringomyelic syndrome (suspended sensory levels)
impairment of all sensory modalities below the level of the transection	impaired light touch, two-point discrimination, vibration and proprioception below the level of the lesion; pain and temperature sensation are preserved	impaired pain and temperature below the level of the lesion; dorsal column modalities spared	impairment of all modalities at site of dorsal root; impaired light touch, two-point discrimination, vibration sense, and proprioception below the level of the lesion and on the same side; impaired pain and temperature sensation on the opposite side	bilateral impairment of pain and temperature in the segments affected by the lesion; dorsal column modalities spared

Fig. 14.3 Distribution of sensory disturbance caused by lesions of the spinal cord.

side within the distribution of the dermatomes affected. "Pyramidal-pattern" weakness is present on the side of the lesion. Examples include tumor deposits and demyelination.

Central cord lesion
A central cord lesion affects the crossing spinothalamic fibers, with sparing of the dorsal columns. There is bilateral loss of pain and temperature perception in the segments affected by the lesion. As the spinothalamic tracts are not involved, the segments above and below the region of the lesion will be spared. Segmental amyotrophy and loss of reflexes may occur from involvement of anterior horn cells and fibers subserving the reflex arc within the cord.

Lesions of the brainstem
Lower medulla
A lesion of the lower medulla (Fig. 14.4) causes impairment of pain and temperature perception of the ipsilateral face and the contralateral body. Light

touch, two-point discrimination, vibration, and proprioception may be impaired on the side of the lesion. Examples include a lateral medullary infarction involving the trigeminal nucleus and crossed spinothalamic tract.

Upper medulla, pons and midbrain
A lesion of the upper medulla, pons, or midbrain causes impairment of all sensory modalities on the opposite side of the body including the face, since all the sensory tracts have already crossed.

The brainstem syndromes discussed above may be accompanied by cranial nerve palsies and cerebellar signs ipsilateral to the lesion, and contralateral hemiparesis.

Lesions of the thalamus
A thalamic lesion (see Fig. 14.4) causes impairment of all sensory modalities on the opposite side of the body including the face. There may be pain of the affected side—the thalamic pain syndrome.

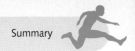

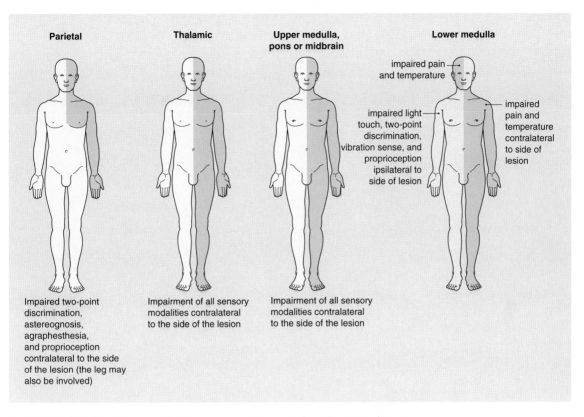

Parietal

Impaired two-point discrimination, astereognosis, agraphesthesia, and proprioception contralateral to the side of the lesion (the leg may also be involved)

Thalamic

Impairment of all sensory modalities contralateral to the side of the lesion

Upper medulla, pons or midbrain

impaired light touch, two-point discrimination, vibration sense, and proprioception ipsilateral to side of lesion

Impairment of all sensory modalities contralateral to the side of the lesion

Lower medulla

impaired pain and temperature

impaired pain and temperature contralateral to side of lesion

Fig. 14.4 Distribution of sensory disturbance caused by cerebral and brainstem lesions.

Lesions of the parietal lobe

A parietal lobe lesion (see Fig. 14.4) causes:

- Loss of discriminative sensory function of the opposite side of the face and limbs—there is impaired two-point discrimination, lack of recognition of objects by touch (astereognosis) or figures drawn on the hand (agraphesthesia), and loss of perception of limb position. However, the primary modalities of pain, temperature, touch, and vibration are intact.
- Sensory inattention—the patient ignores all stimuli on the opposite side of the body when the stimulus is applied bilaterally. However, when applied on the affected side only, the sensory examination is normal. This neglect also occurs when testing the visual fields. The lesion is usually of the nondominant parietal cortex.

A dissociated pattern of sensory loss between the modalities of pain and temperature and those of light touch, two-point discrimination, vibration, and proprioception occurs in:
- Central cord lesions.
- Hemisection of the cord.
- Lateral medullary lesions.

Summary

Typical patterns of sensory impairment resulting from central and peripheral lesions are shown in Figs 14.2–14.4.

15. Disorders of Gait

The character of a patient's gait will provide clues to the clinical signs that may be expected on further neurologic examination. When assessing a patient's gait, the following categories should be kept in mind:
- Cerebellar ataxia.
- Spastic.
- Hemiparetic.
- Parkinsonian.
- Sensory ataxia.
- Steppage.
- Myopathic.
- Apraxic.
- Antalgic.
- Psychogenic.

If the gait is characteristic of one of the above, this will be confirmed by further neurologic examination. A differential diagnosis of the etiology can then be made with clues obtained from the history and examination.

The main gait disorders are illustrated in Fig. 15.1.

Differential diagnosis

Gait of cerebellar ataxia

Patients with cerebellar ataxia stand and walk on a wide-based gait, i.e., with feet spaced widely apart (Fig. 15.1A). The gait is unsteady, with irregularity of stride. The trunk sways, and the patient may veer towards one side. In mild cases the only manifestation of gait disturbance may be difficulty in walking heel-to-toe in a straight line (i.e., tandem-walking). Note that Romberg's test is usually normal.

Look for cerebellar signs in the limbs; these may be unilateral or bilateral. Ataxia of gait may be the only sign of cerebellar dysfunction, particularly with a midline lesion.

Causes include:
- Multiple sclerosis.
- Alcoholic cerebellar degeneration.
- Antiepileptic drug therapy.
- Posterior fossa tumors.
- Cerebellar paraneoplastic syndrome.
- The hereditary cerebellar ataxias.

Hemiparetic gait

In patients who have a hemiparetic gait, firstly note the characteristic posture on one side, i.e., flexion of the upper limb and extension of the lower limb (Fig. 15.1B; see also Fig. 13.2). The latter moves stiffly and is swung round in a semicircle to avoid scraping the foot across the floor. However, such scraping does occur to some extent and the toe and outer sole of the shoe become worn.

Causes include:
- Cerebral hemisphere stroke.
- Neoplastic infiltration.
- Traumatic lesion.

Spastic gait

A spastic gait is seen in patients who have a spastic paraparesis or bilateral hemiparesis. The legs move slowly and stiffly; the thighs are strongly adducted such that the legs may cross as the patient walks (scissor gait).

Causes include:
- Spinal cord compression.
- Trauma—spinal surgery.
- Birth injuries or congenital deformities—cerebral palsy, spina bifida.
- Multiple sclerosis.
- Motor neuron disease.
- Parasagittal meningioma.
- Subacute combined degeneration of the cord.

Parkinsonian gait

With parkinsonian gait, note the stooped posture and loss of arm swing, which may be more marked on one side (Fig. 15.1C; also see Fig. 23.4). The steps are short, and the patient shuffles. There may be difficulty starting, stopping, or turning.

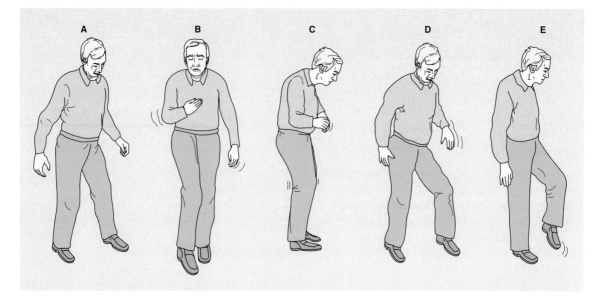

Fig. 15.1 Disorders of gait. (A) Cerebellar ataxia, (B) hemiparetic, (C) parkinsonian, (D) sensory ataxia, and (E) unilateral footdrop.

Having started to walk, the patient leans forward and the pace quickens, as though the patient is attempting to catch up on himself or herself (festinating) gait.

Gait of sensory ataxia

Sensory ataxia arises from impaired proprioception caused by a lesion of the peripheral nerves, posterior roots, dorsal columns in the spinal cord, or rarely the ascending afferent fibers to the parietal lobes. The gait is "stomping" (Fig. 15.1D). Romberg's test is positive and there is impaired perception of joint position on examination of the lower limbs. Shoe soles are equally worn throughout.

Causes include:
- Posterior spinal cord lesions.
- Vitamin B_{12} deficiency.
- Tabes dorsalis (syphilis).
- Cervical spondylosis.
- Multiple sclerosis.
- Tumors.

Sensory peripheral neuropathies include:
- Hereditary—Charcot–Marie–Tooth disease.
- Metabolic—diabetes.
- Inflammatory—Guillain Barré syndrome.
- Malignancy—myeloma, paraneoplastic syndrome.
- Toxic—alcohol, drugs (e.g., isoniazid).

Steppage gait

Steppage gait arises from weakness of the tibial and peroneal muscles of lower motor neuron type. The patient has "footdrop" and is unable to dorsiflex and evert the foot (Fig. 15.1E). The leg is lifted high on walking so that the toes clear the ground. On striking the floor again, there is a slapping noise. Shoe soles are worn on the anterior and lateral aspects.

Causes include:
- Charcot–Marie–Tooth disease (bilateral footdrop).
- Lateral popliteal nerve palsy (e.g., from a fibular fracture [unilateral footdrop]).
- Anterior horn cell disease (e.g., polio, motor neuron disease [often asymmetrical footdrop]).

Myopathic gait

Myopathic gait is the so-called waddling gait caused by weakness of the proximal muscles of the lower limb girdle. The weight is alternately placed on each leg, with the opposite hip and side of the trunk tilting up towards the weight-bearing side; however, the weak gluteal muscles cannot stabilize the weight-bearing hip, which sways outward, with the opposite pelvis dropping, as does the trunk on that side.

Causes include:
- Muscular dystrophies—Duchenne's, Becker's, limb-girdle, facioscapulohumeral.

- Metabolic myopathies—periodic paralysis, hypo- and hyperkalemia, hypo- and hypercalcemia.
- Endocrine myopathies—Cushing's disease, Addison's disease, hypo- and hyperthyroidism.
- Inflammatory myopathies—polymyositis and dermatomyositis.

Apraxic gait

Disease of the frontal lobes gives rise to an apraxic gait. The patient walks with feet placed apart, and with small, hesitant steps, which may be described as "walking on ice." There is difficulty with initiation of walking, and with advanced cases it may seem as though the patient's feet are stuck to the floor. Notably there is no abnormality of power, sensation, or coordination. Look for signs of frontal cortical dysfunction (e.g., a grasp or snout reflex); the tendon reflexes may be brisk and the plantar responses extensor.

Causes include:
- Bilateral subcortical cerebrovascular disease.
- Normal-pressure hydrocephalus.
- Frontal lobe tumors (e.g., meningioma).
- Frontal subdural hematomas (rare; bilateral usually).
- Alzheimer's dementia.

Antalgic gait

Antalgic gait arises from pain (e.g., a painful hip or knee due to arthritis). The patient tends to weight-bear mainly on the unaffected side, only briefly putting weight onto the affected side; thus the tendency to hobble.

Psychogenic gait

Psychogenic gait does not conform to any of the descriptions given above. It may take a number of forms and is variable in character. There are no objective abnormal neurological signs on formal examination. Note, however, that the only manifestation of a midline cerebellar lesion may be severe ataxia of gait and stance, with normal limb signs on formal examination.

The character of a patient's gait will provide clues to the clinical signs that might be expected on further neurologic examination:
- Ataxic—wide based and unsteady.
- Hemiplegic—unilateral flexed posture of the upper limb and extended posture of the lower limb.
- Spastic—"scissoring" posture of the legs.
- Parkinsonian—stooped posture, shuffling small stepped gait with loss of arm swing.
- Sensory ataxia—high stepped, "stomping" gait.
- Steppage—footdrop.
- Myopathic—"waddling" gait.
- Apraxic—hesitant, "walking-on-ice" gait.
- Psychogenic—bizarre and variable.

HISTORY, EXAMINATION, AND COMMON INVESTIGATIONS

16. Taking a History

Things to remember when taking a history

Taking a history is the most important part of the assessment of a patient with neurologic symptoms. Many common conditions, such as headache and epilepsy, are diagnosed from the clinical history.

General observation of the patient as he or she walks into the examination room or as you approach the bed is important:
- Does the patient appear unwell?
- Does he or she use any aids (canes, crutches, walker, wheelchair, hearing-aid)?
- Are there any obvious morphologic abnormalities (e.g., weakness on one side, drooping of the face, wasting of the muscles, involuntary movements, abnormal gait)?

The initial approach is important to establish rapport:
- Introduce yourself.
- Explain who you are.
- Ask if you may talk to and examine him or her.
- Ask age and occupation.
- Ask whether he or she is right- or left-handed (if you do not ask this at the beginning, you may forget).

Quite quickly you should be able to make some inferences about the patient's mood and cognitive state:
- Does the patient respond appropriately (indicating probable preservation of important higher mental functioning)?
- Does he or she appear to be depressed (which may be part of the patient's neurologic condition or may indicate a reaction to it) or elated (as in patients who have frontal lobe dysfunction)?
- Is the patient's speech normal?

Structure of the history

The chief complaint (CC)
Consider the CC from the patient's point of view. Ask:
- "What is the main problem?"
- "What was it that caused you to go to your doctor/come to the hospital?"

When presenting the history to others, use the patient's language (e.g., "This woman complains of seeing double")—not the medical terminology (e.g., "This woman complains of horizontal diplopia").

History of the presenting illness (HPI)
Establish the HPI by asking:
- When it was first noted by the patient.
- Was the onset sudden, subacute, or insidious and gradual?
- Is the symptom episodic or constant?
- Has it worsened, improved, or stayed the same since?
- What is its nature (e.g., headache may be throbbing, stabbing or pressure-like) and its distribution (e.g., unilateral, bilateral, frontal, occipital)?
- Is there anything that makes it better (e.g., medicines, sleep, exercise) or worse (e.g., movement, coughing, posture)?
- Are there any associated symptoms (e.g., vomiting, photophobia, neck stiffness)?
- Have any other symptoms developed since this first complaint was noticed (in particular additional neurologic symptoms such as blurred vision or unsteady gait)?
- Has the patient ever had other neurologic symptoms in the past? These may be related. For example, an episode of transient visual loss 5 years

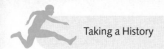

previously in a young woman now complaining of difficulty in walking is indicative of possible multiple sclerosis.

- Have any tests already been performed? If so, where and when?

Further questions pertaining to the HPI will relate to the differential diagnosis of the main complaint, the most common of which are outlined in Part I.

Past medical history (PMH)

Some clinicians prefer to take the PMH before considering the presenting complaint, because there may be important background information. The following may be relevant in neurologic cases:

- Birth and early development.
- Infections during childhood.
- Head injuries.
- Hypertension, ischemic heart disease, rheumatic fever.
- Diabetes.
- A systemic disorder (e.g., systemic lupus erythematosus).

Review of systems (ROS)

Review the following body systems:

- Gastrointestinal: appetite, weight loss or gain, swallowing, change in bowel function.
- Cardiovascular: chest pain, shortness of breath, palpitations, claudication.
- Respiratory: cough, shortness of breath.
- Genitourinary: bladder function, impotence, sexual function.
- Musculoskeletal: joint pain, stiffness.
- Skin: rash, birthmarks.
- Mood.
- Memory.
- Endocrine: menses, heat/cold tolerance.
- General: sleep.

Drug history (DH)

To determine the DH, find out from the patient:

- Is he or she taking any medicines now, or have any been taken for some time in the past?
- Are there any known drug allergies?

Family history (FH)

To determine the FH, find out from the patient:

- Are there any "family illnesses"?
- Are parents, siblings, and children alive and well? If not, what did they die from and at what age?

Social history (SH)

To determine the SH, ask the patient about:

- Occupation.
- Home circumstances: with whom the patient lives, own home, stairs, social-service help.
- Smoking history.
- Alcohol intake (drinks/week)—is there a past history of heavy alcohol consumption?
- Diet (vegetarian or vegan).
- Sexual history or orientation—this may be relevant in certain cases.

Summary

When presenting the history, run through the categories described above, always starting with the same pattern (e.g., "Ms. Randolph is a 40-year-old right-handed administrator who complains of numbness in the feet").

Describe the HPI, PMH, and ROS. You do not have to mention specifically all negative points, but it is worth pointing out those that are important (e.g., "She has no history of diabetes").

Say whether the patient is taking any medication.

Describe the FH if relevant; if not, state "There is no relevant family history".

Describe important social points (e.g., "She drinks only moderate amounts of alcohol and has never smoked").

You will then move on to your examination findings.

When presenting the history, always start with the same sequence:
- Name.
- Age.
- Handedness, if relevant.
- Occupation.
- Complaint (in the patient's words).

Then continue with:
- History of presenting illness.
- Past medical history.
- Medication history.
- Family history.
- Social history.
- Review of systems.

17. The Neurologic Examination

Mental status and higher cerebral functions

Consciousness

Consciousness is the state of being aware of self and the environment. A number of ill-defined terms are used to describe different levels of arousal:

- Alert—full wakefulness and immediate and appropriate responsiveness. The patient is orientated to person, time, and place.
- Lethargic—the inability to think with usual speed and clarity. There may be lack of attention, disorientation in time and place, and impairment of memory.
- Obtundation—the patient is drowsy and indifferent to the environment but responsive to verbal stimuli.
- Stupor—the patient is unconscious but arousable when stimulated.
- Coma—the patient is unaware of self and the environment and is not arousable.

The level of consciousness is more objectively assessed using the Glasgow Coma Scale (see Fig. 2.2).

Appearance and behavior

Assessment of the patient's mental state begins as soon as you meet the patient. The physical appearance can be helpful. Demented patients may look bewildered but unconcerned or apathetic and withdrawn. Look for evidence of self-neglect, which is often concealed by relatives. Observe the patient's response to your questions during the history taking, assessing his or her comprehension and whether he or she retains insight into his or her problem.

Affect

Note the patient's affect.

- Does the patient seem depressed?
- Loss of interest, euphoria, or social disinhibition may be signs of frontal lobe dysfunction. Emotional behavior such as aggression and anger may arise from damage to the limbic system.

- Emotional lability should prompt further examination to look for upper motor neuron signs and a pseudobulbar palsy.

Cognitive function
Mini-mental state examination

The mini-mental state examination is a screening test for several different cognitive (intellectual) functions (Fig. 17.1):

- Orientation of person, time, and place establishes full awareness of self and the environment. Further testing requires the patient to be alert.
- Registration and recall assess short-term memory. Remote memory may be tested by asking about memories of childhood, work, or marriage. These need corroboration. Verbal memory may be tested by asking the patient to remember a sentence or short story and to recall it 15 minutes later. Visual memory can be assessed by asking the patient to memorize three objects and recall them after 5 minutes.
- Attention and calculation can be tested by asking the patient to spell a five-letter word backward and to subtract 7 from 100 and continue to subtract 7 from each answer obtained; if the latter is too complex for the patient's premorbid calculation skills, simple arithmetic can be used.
- Language examination tests comprehension of speech and written language and includes tests for aphasia, dyslexia, dysgraphia, and constructional ability.

The maximum score is 30. Scores of less than 25 suggest the presence of cognitive impairment. Formal psychometric testing should be performed for all patients suspected of having impaired cognition.

Dyspraxia and apraxia

Apraxia is inability and dyspraxia is difficulty performing skilled movement in the absence of weakness, sensory loss, incoordination, or impaired comprehension. Apraxia and dyspraxia arise from a lesion of the nondominant parietal cortex. The

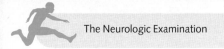

Mini-mental state examination

Orientation
1. What is the year, season, date, month, day? (one point for each correct answer)
2. Where are we? Country, county, town, hospital, floor? (one point for each answer)

Registration
3. Name three objects, taking 1 second to say each. Then ask the patient to name all three. One point for each correct answer. Repeat the question until the patient learns all three

Attention and calculation
4. Serial sevens. One point for each correct answer. Stop after five answers Alternative: spell "WORLD" backward

Recall
5. Ask for names of the three objects asked in question 3. One point for each correct answer

Language
6. Point to a pencil and a watch. Ask the patient to name them for you. One point for each correct answer
7. Ask the patient to repeat "No ifs, ands, or buts". One point
8. Ask the patient to follow a three-stage command: "Take the paper in your right hand; fold the paper in half; put the paper on the floor." Three points
9. Ask the patient to read and obey the following: CLOSE YOUR EYES (Write this in large letters.) One point
10. Ask the patient to write a sentence of his or her own choice. (The sentence must contain a subject and an object and make some sense.) Ignore spelling errors when scoring. One point
11. Ask the patient to copy two intersecting pentagons with equal sides. Give one point if all the sides and angles are preserved and if the intersecting sides form a quadrangle

Maximum score = 30 points

Fig. 17.1 The mini-mental state test.

ability to perform skilled tasks can be tested as follows:
- Upper limbs—the patient's ability to use a pen or comb can be assessed. Dressing can be assessed by asking the patient to put on a shirt.
- Lower limbs—the ability to walk can be tested by examining the gait (see p. 83).
- Face—the patient is asked to "blow a kiss" or to whistle.

Agnosia
Agnosia is the failure to appreciate the significance of a sensory stimulus without the aid of other senses in the presence of intact peripheral sensation (tactile, visual, and auditory). There are different types:
- Tactile agnosia (or astereognosis) is the inability to recognize a familiar object placed in the hand with eyes closed and silence (e.g., patients cannot recognize keys placed in the palm of their hand without looking at them or hearing them rattle). It arises from a lesion of the contralateral posterior parietal lobe.
- Visual agnosia is the inability to recognize a familiar object by looking at it without touching it or hearing any sound from it (e.g., a telephone). It arises from a lesion of the (usually dominant) parieto-occipital lobe.
- Auditory agnosia is the inability to recognize a sound such as a bell ringing without seeing or feeling the bell. It arises from a lesion of the dominant temporal lobe.

Clinical syndromes associated with specific focal hemispheric dysfunction
Frontal lobe
Patients who have a lesion of the frontal lobe should be tested for the following:

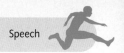

- A contralateral mono- or hemiparesis and lower facial weakness (see pp. 43–44 and 68).
- Broca's aphasia (see p. 3).
- Behavioral change—alteration in personality or mood and loss of interest and initiative can be observed by watching the patient and through conversation.
- Loss of abstract thought—can be tested by the patient's interpretation of proverbs (e.g., people that live in glass houses should not throw stones) and by the patient's ability to identify similarities between pairs of objects (e.g., cow and dog, chair and table).
- Primitive reflexes—the grasp reflex is usually found in infants and consists of flexion of the thumb and fingers on stroking the skin of the palm. The sucking and snout reflexes can be elicited by lightly stroking the lips, which produces a sucking response, and tapping the closed lips, which causes the snout reflex.
- Apraxia of gait (see p. 83 and Chapter 15).

Parietal lobe

Features of a lesion of the dominant parietal lobe are:
- Contralateral discriminatory sensory impairment—impairment of position sense and two-point discrimination and inability to recognize objects by form and texture (astereognosis) or figures drawn on the hand (agraphasthesia). Pain, temperature, touch, and vibration sensation are intact, but their localization when applied to the body may be impaired.
- Visual field deficit—contralateral lower homonymous quadrantanopia
- Right–left disorientation.
- Finger agnosia—the inability to recognize and identify the fingers of the hand correctly.
- Dyscalculia— calculation is impaired when asked to perform serial sevens or simple arithmetic.
- Dyslexia—difficulty with reading.
- Ideomotor and ideational dyspraxia—difficulty in carrying out a task on request or by imitation.

Features of a lesion of the nondominant parietal lobe are:
- Constructional apraxia—the patient has difficulty drawing a simple object or with constructing an object, e.g. using building blocks.
- Dressing apraxia—the patient has difficulty putting on and taking off clothes.

- Contralateral sensory inattention—the patient neglects the opposite side of the body. This may be sensory, motor, or visual. Sensory inattention can be tested by asking patients to close their eyes and for the examiner to touch their right or left leg (or arm or face), then to touch both sides together. These patients will identify touch on each side individually, but when touched on both sides will only identify touch on the side of the lesion, neglecting the contralateral side. Visual inattention may be similarly elicited by testing the visual fields (see pp. 93–94) ; these patients will have normal visual fields when each side is tested individually, but when both visual fields are tested the side contralateral to the lesion will be neglected. A hemiplegic patient may ignore the paralyzed side of the body.

Temporal lobe

Patients who have a lesion of the temporal lobe should be tested for the following:
- Wernicke's aphasia (see p. 6).
- Auditory agnosia (see p. 90).
- Visual field deficit—there is a contralateral upper homonymous quadrantanopia.
- Learning difficulties and memory impairment—bilateral lesions result in impaired retention of new information.
- Emotional disturbances—aggression, rage, and change in sexual function.

Occipital lobe

Patients who have a lesion of the occipital lobe should be tested for the following:
- Visual field deficit—there may be a contralateral homonymous hemianopia (note that a lesion of posterior cerebral artery spares the macula and a lesion of the occipital pole results in a contralateral macular homonymous hemianopic field defect); bilateral occipital lesions render the patient blind, but with normal pupillary reflexes.
- Visual agnosia (see p. 90).

Speech

Speech production is organized at three levels:
- Phonation.
- Articulation.
- Language production.

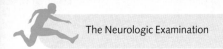

Phonation

Phonation is the production of sounds as the air passes through the vocal cords. A disorder of this process is called dysphonia.

Assessment

Speech will have already been heard during the history taking. In dysphonia, the speech volume is reduced and the voice may sound hoarse or husky.

Aphonia is the inability to produce sound. Coughing may be impaired because this requires normal vocal cord function. Therefore, the ability to cough should be tested.

Articulation

Articulation is the manipulation of sound as it passes through the upper airways by the palate, the tongue, and the lips to produce phonemes. A disorder of this process is called dysarthria.

Assessment

To assess articulation, ask patients a series of questions such as their name and address and, for longer answers, what they had for breakfast or have done that morning. Ask patients to repeat a series of phrases—"baby hippopotamus," "Methodist Episcopal," "American constitution." From this the characteristics of the speech can be gained and then localization of the site of the lesion, confirmed by additional neurologic signs on formal examination (see Chapter 10). Always look for a local lesion of the oropharynx first.

Dysarthria may result from a lesion of the:
- Upper motor neuron (pseudobulbar palsy)—slow, high-pitched and forced.
- Lower motor neuron (bulbar palsy)—slurred and indistinct with nasal intonation; labial and lingual sounds are affected.
- Basal ganglia—rapidly spoken words, low-pitched, and monotonous (akinetic–rigid syndromes); loud, harsh, and with variable intonation (chorea and myoclonus); loud, slow, and indistinct consonants (athetoid).
- Cerebellum—slow and slurred, scanning or staccato quality if there is also involvement of the corticobulbar tracts.
- Muscle and neuromuscular junction—the characteristics of the dysarthria are similar to those of a bulbar palsy. There may be a deterioration in the quality of speech (fatiguability) in Myasthenia Gravis.

Language production

Language production is the organization of phonemes into words and sentences, and is controlled by the speech centers in the dominant hemisphere (Broca's and Wernicke's areas). A disorder of this process is called aphasia.

Assessment

To assess language production:
- Establish the patient's handedness. Aphasia is a feature of dominant-hemisphere dysfunction. The left hemisphere is dominant in over 90% of right-handed and about 60% of left-handed individuals.
- Listen to the patient's spontaneous speech, assessing its fluency and content.
- Assess the patient's comprehension by observing his or her response to simple commands (e.g., "Open your mouth," "Look up to the ceiling").
- Assess the patient's ability to name objects. Use your wristwatch (face, hands, strap, buckle).
- Assess the patient's ability to repeat sentences (e.g., "No ifs, ands, or buts").

An expressive dysphasia arises from a lesion of Broca's area. The speech is nonfluent and hesitant, but comprehension is intact. Repetition is better than spontaneous speech. The patient has difficulty finding the correct words and often produces an incorrect word (paraphrasia). Such patients retain insight into their language disturbance.

A receptive aphasia arises from a lesion of Wernicke's area. The speech is fluent, but the words are partly correct, incorrect but related to the intended word (paraphrasia), or newly created (neologisms). The language is therefore unintelligible, but the patient is unaware of the problem.

Anomia is the inability to name objects. It can occur following recovery from other types of dysphasia.

The clinical features of the different types of dysphasia are summarized in Fig. 17.2.

The cranial nerves

Introduction

Examination of the cranial nerves plays an important part in the assessment of the central nervous system. It aids lesion localization and has important prognostic implications in the unconscious patient.

Classification of aphasia					
Type	Lesion	Speech fluency	Speech content	Comprehension	Repetition
expressive	Broca's area	nonfluent	normal	normal	variable
anomia	angular gyrus	fluent	normal	normal	normal
receptive	Wernicke's area	fluent	impaired	impaired	impaired
conductive	arcuate fasciculus	fluent	impaired	normal	impaired
global	frontal, parietal, and temporal lobe	nonfluent	impaired	impaired	impaired

Fig. 17.2 Classification of aphasia.

Olfactory (first) nerve

To test the olfactory nerve, first ask the patient about any recent change in their sense of smell. A characteristic-smelling object (e.g., peppermint, clove oil) is held under each nostril in turn while the other is occluded and the patient keeps the eyes closed. An individual who has intact olfaction can detect the smell, and discriminate and name it. The recommended special testing bottles are rarely available when needed and most clinicians perform preliminary assessment with nearby objects such as fruit, a coffee jar, or gum. Avoid using irritating odors (e.g., ammonia or camphor), which will stimulate the trigeminal nerve.

Unilateral loss of smell is usually asymptomatic. Bilateral loss of smell may be associated with an altered sensation of taste (loss of the ability to appreciate aromas) (dysguesia or aguesia).

When examining patients who have anosmia it is important to look carefully for frontal lobe signs and evidence of optic nerve or chiasmal damage. More often there will be pathology in the nasal passages or sinuses.

Optic (second) nerve
Visual acuity

Visual acuity (VA) is tested using a Snellen chart in a well-lit room. Seat or stand the patient 20 feet from the chart. Small, hand-held Snellen charts can be read at a distance of 14 inches from the eye. Near VA is tested using reading charts, but this does not necessarily correlate with distance acuity.

Correct the patient's refractive error with glasses or a pinhole. Ask the patient to cover each eye in turn with his or her palm, and find which line of print he or she can read comfortably. VA is expressed as the ratio of the distance between the patient and the chart to the number of the smallest visible line on the chart (normally 20/20) (Fig. 17.3).

If the patient is unable to read characters of line 800 (VA less than 20/800), assess his or her ability to count your fingers at 3 feet (VA:CF), see your hand movements (VA:HM), or perceive a light (VA:PL). If unable to perceive light (VA:NPL), the patient is blind.

Color vision

Color vision is tested using Ishihara plates in a daylight-lit room. Test each eye separately. If at least 13 out of 15 plates are read correctly, color vision can be regarded as normal.

This test is designed principally to detect congenital color vision defects but is sensitive in detecting mild degrees of optic nerve dysfunction.

Visual fields

Sit about 3 feet from the patient with your eyes at the same horizontal level. Start by testing for visual inattention. Ask the patient to look into your eyes; hold your hands halfway between you and the patient. Stimulate the patient's visual fields by moving each hand separately and then both hands together, and ask the patient to indicate which of your hands has moved each time.

In patients with a nondominant parietal lobe lesion, a visual stimulus presented in isolation to the contralateral field is perceived, but it may be missed when a comparable stimulus is presented simultaneously to the ipsilateral field.

Visual fields are examined by confrontation, during which you compare your own visual fields

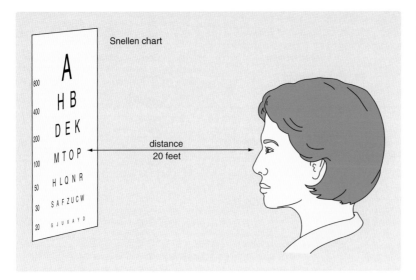

Fig. 17.3 Visual acuity. The patient is able to read line number 100 but not line number 50. Visual acuity is 20/100.

with the patient's on the assumption that yours are normal. The patient's visual field will match yours only if your head positions are exactly comparable and if your hand is exactly halfway between you and the patient.

Visual fields in poorly cooperative patients are assessed by the response to visual threat (sudden, unexpected hand movement into the patient's visual field).

Peripheral fields

Examine each eye in turn. To test the patient's right visual field, ask the patient to cover his or her left eye with his or her left palm and to look into your left eye throughout the examination.

Cover your right eye with your right hand, and test the patient's peripheral field by bringing the moving fingers of your left hand into the upper and then the lower quadrants of the patient's temporal fields. Ask the patient to inform you as soon as he or she sees your fingers.

Now cover your right eye with your left hand and examine the patient's nasal fields with your right hand, using the same method.

Lesions of different parts of the visual pathway produce characteristic field defects (see Fig. 5.2) and are discussed in Chapter 5.

Blind spot

Routine testing is unnecessary, but enlargement of the blind spot may be an important finding in patients with raised intracranial pressure.

The blind spot is tested using a 10-mm red pin. Ask the patient to cover his or her left eye, and move the pin from the central into the temporal field, along the horizontal meridian, having explained to the patient that the pin will disappear briefly and then reappear again, and that he or she should indicate when this happens. Once you have found the patient's blind spot, you can map its shape and compare its size with yours.

Central field

The central field is tested by moving a red pin along the central visual field (fixation area), in the horizontal meridian. Ask the patient to indicate if the pin disappears (absolute central scotoma) or if the color appears diminished (relative scotoma). A central scotoma may extend temporally from the fixation area into the blind spot (centrocecal scotoma).

Perimetry

Peripheral visual fields are sensitive to a moving target and formally tested with Goldmann perimetry. The patient fixates on a central point and a point of light moves centrally from the periphery. The patient indicates the position of the point of light each time and this is plotted on a chart. Repetitive testing from different directions accurately records the visual fields. Central fields can be tested using this method, but with a less intense light source. Humphrey fields use a static light source. A record of the threshold of the light source with increasing intensity provides information about the central visual field.

Fundoscopy

Ask the patient to fixate on a distant target, best done in dimmed light. Using a direct ophthalmoscope, examine the patient's right eye using your right eye, and the patient's left eye using your left eye.

Adjust the ophthalmoscope lens until the retinal vessels are in focus, and trace them back to the optic disc. Assess the shape and color of the optic disc and the clarity of its margins. The temporal disc margins are normally slightly paler than the nasal margins. The physiologic cupping varies in size but does not extend to the disc margins.

Next, assess the retinal vessels. The arteries are narrower than the veins and brighter in color. The vessels should not be obscured as they cross the disc margins. Look for retinal vein pulsation, which is present in about 80% of normal individuals and is an index of normal intracranial pressure. This is seen best at the disc margins where the veins cross over the arteries. Note the width of the blood vessels and look for arteriovenous nicking at the crossover points.

Assess the rest of the retina, noting any evidence of discoloration, hemorrhages, or white patches of exudate. Ask the patient to look at the light of the ophthalmoscope, which brings the macula into view. Classify fundoscopic abnormalities into those affecting the optic disc, the retinal vessels, or the retina (Fig. 17.4).

Oculomotor (third), trochlear (fourth), and abducens (sixth) nerves
Eyelids

Ptosis is drooping of the upper eyelid and is most often partial. A full ptosis (complete closure of the eyelid) is usually due to a third nerve palsy. Examination of pupil responses and eye movements provide essential information about the cause of the ptosis (Fig. 17.5).

Pupils

Assess the size and shape of the pupils. They should be circular and symmetrical (see Fig. 6.3).

Light response

Light responses should be assessed using a bright light. Ask the patient to fixate on a distant target, and shine the light into each eye in turn, shining light quickly onto the pupil from the lateral side. Observe the direct (ipsilateral) and the consensual (contralateral) responses.

Assess the presence of an afferent pupillary defect by swinging the light from one eye to the other, dwelling 3 seconds on each. As you swing the light from the right eye to the left, the pupil of the latter (which has just started to dilate because of loss of its consensual reaction) should immediately constrict. A delayed or incomplete constriction indicates loss of sensitivity of the afferent pathway in that eye (optic nerve damage).

Accommodation

Hold your finger 2 feet from the patient and ask him or her to fixate on it. Bring your finger towards the patient's eyes. Observe for the normal reaction of bilateral pupillary constriction and convergence (adduction).

Eye movements

Inspect the eyes and note the position of the eyelids and the presence of any strabismus (misalignment of the visual axes) (see pp. 35–36).

If the patient is capable of voluntary eye movements, the pursuit and saccadic systems should be tested to assess whether eye movements are conjugate, and to detect the presence of diplopia and nystagmus:

Pursuit eye movements

Hold the index finger of your hand 2 feet in front of the patient's eyes. Ask the patient to follow your slowly moving finger throughout the range of binocular vision in both horizontal and vertical planes in an "H" pattern.

Assess the smoothness, speed, and magnitude of the movements. Look for nystagmus, and ask the patient to report any diplopia. In the presence of diplopia, identify the direction of the maximum separation of images and the two muscles responsible for moving the eyes in this direction (see Fig. 6.4). Identify the source of the outer image, which comes from the defective eye, by covering each eye in turn. This will allow you to name the muscle(s) and the nerve(s) involved.

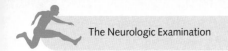

Common fundoscopic abnormalities		
Structure	**Abnormality**	**Pathology**
optic disc	papilledema—the optic disc is "swollen" with blurring of the disc margin and engorgement of the retinal veins; there may be flame-shaped hemorrhages and "cotton wool spots" on or near the disc	raised intracranial pressure (space-occupying lesions, e.g. tumors, particularly of the posterior fossa, hydrocephalus subsequent to meningitis or subarachnoid hemorrhage), venous obstruction (e.g. cavernous sinus thrombosis), malignant hypertension, idiopathic intracranial hypertension
	optic atrophy—the optic disc of patients who have acute optic neuritis may have an appearance similar to that of papilledema, but in acute optic neuritis eye movements can be painful and visual acuity is substantially reduced	central retinal artery occlusion, optic neuritis (multiple sclerosis, ischemia), chronic glaucoma, B_{12} deficiency, toxins (e.g. methyl alcohol, tobacco), hereditary (e.g. Leber's optic atrophy), lesion of the optic chiasm and or tract
retinal arteries	silver-wiring, increased tortuosity, arteriovenous nicking	hypertension
	gross narrowing with retinal pallor and reddened fovea	central retinal artery occlusion
	cholesterol or platelet emboli	cerebrovascular disease
	new vessel formation (on the surface of the optic disc or retinal): new vessels develop subsequent to widespread retinal ischemia; they do not affect vision, but are fragile and may bleed	diabetes, central or branch retinal vein occlusion
retinal veins	venous engorgement	papilledema (see above), central retinal vein occlusion
retina	hemorrhages	superficial flame-shaped and deep dot-shaped (hypertension, diabetes, subhyaloid between the retina and the vitreous (subarachnoid hemorrhage)
	exudates	"soft cotton-wool spots" (retinal infarcts) and hard exudates (lipid accumulation within the retina from leaking blood vessels in hypertension and diabetes)
	pigmentation	retinitis pigmentosa (e.g. Refsum's disease, Kearns–Sayre syndrome), choroidoretinitis (e.g. toxoplasmosis, sarcoidosis, syphilis), postlaser treatment (diabetes)

Fig. 17.4 Common fundoscopic abnormalities.

Saccadic eye movements

Ask the patient to keep his or her head still, and to look left, right, up, and down as quickly as possible. Assess the velocity and the accuracy of the movements. Look for slow or absent adduction (internuclear ophthalmoplegia: see Fig. 6.9).

If pursuit or saccadic eye movements are absent, the oculocephalic reflex (doll's eye movements) will differentiate between supranuclear and nuclear ocular paralysis. Ask the patient to fixate on your eyes while you rotate his or her head in the horizontal and the vertical planes. In supranuclear lesions, the reflex is intact, allowing the patient's eyes to remain fixated on yours.

Ocular nerve paresis

Clinical signs and causes of ocular nerve paresis are discussed in Chapter 6.

Nystagmus

Nystagmus is an involuntary rhythmic oscillation of the eyes caused by lesions affecting brainstem vertical and horizontal gaze centres and their vestibular and cerebellar connections. It is usually asymptomatic but patients sometimes describe oscillopsia, an unpleasant experience of alternating movements of their visual fields.

Nystagmus must be differentiated from end-point nystagmoid jerks seen at extreme deviation of gaze,

Assessment of ptosis			
Cause	Additional clinical features	Pupil responses	Eye movements
Congenital	hereditary; unilateral or bilateral	normal	normal
Neurogenic 3rd nerve palsy (see p. 36 and Fig. 6.6)	complete ptosis	dilated pupil, absent response to light and accommodation	ophthalmoplegia with diplopia in all positions of gaze
Horner's syndrome	partial ptosis, apparent enophthalmos; ipsilateral anhidrosis	constricted pupil, impaired response to light and accommodation	normal
Myogenic senile	this is due to degenerative changes in the levator superioris muscle of the upper eyelid	normal; senile pupil—constricted with impaired dilatation in the dark	normal
Myasthenia Gravis	fatiguable and therefore variable ptosis	normal	variable diplopia and ophthalmoplegia

Fig. 17.5 Assessment of ptosis.

and from the voluntary rapid oscillation of eyes. Both are brief and unsustained.

Note the presence of nystagmus in the primary position of gaze (when looking forward) and while examining eye movements, and decide whether it is pendular or jerky, and whether the movements are horizontal, vertical, rotatory, or of mixed nature.

Record its amplitude (fine, medium, coarse) and persistence, and the direction of gaze in which it occurs (the direction of nystagmus is, by convention, the direction of the fast component). Causes of nystagmus are shown in Fig. 17.6.

Trigeminal (fifth) nerve
Motor
Inspect for wasting of the temporalis muscles, which produces hollowing above the zygoma. Ask the patient to clench his or her teeth together, and palpate the masseters, noting any wasting. The pterygoid muscles are assessed by resisting the patient's attempts to open his or her mouth. In unilateral trigeminal lesions, the lower jaw deviates to the paralytic side as the mouth is opened.

Jaw jerk
Jaw jerk is a brainstem stretch reflex. Ask the patient to open his or her mouth slightly. Rest your index finger on the apex of the jaw and tap it with the reflex hammer. The normal response, mouth closure, is due to a reflex contraction of the pterygoid muscles. An absent reflex is not significant, but the reflex becomes pathologically brisk with upper motor neuron lesions.

Sensory
Sensory testing is performed using the same techniques as described on p. 107. Test light touch, pin prick, and temperature over the forehead, the medial aspects of the cheeks, and the chin, which correspond to the ophthalmic, maxillary, and mandibular branches of the trigeminal nerve, respectively (see Fig. 7.1). A partial loss can be detected by comparing the response to the same stimulus on different areas of the face. The clinical pattern of sensory loss depends on the anatomical site of the lesion (Fig. 17.7).

Corneal response is elicited by lightly touching the cornea (not the conjunctiva) with a wisp of cotton. Synchronous blinking of both eyes should occur. An afferent defect (fifth cranial nerve lesion) results in depression or absence of the direct and consensual reflex. An efferent defect (seventh cranial nerve lesion) results in an impairment or absence of the reflex on the side of the facial weakness.

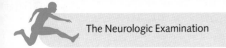

Causes of nystagmus		
Type	**Description**	**Pathology**
pendular	oscillations of equal velocity	longstanding impaired macular vision (since early childhood), e.g., albinism, congenital cataracts
jerky	fast phase towards the side of the lesion	unilateral cerebellar lesions
	fast phase to the opposite side of the lesion	unilateral vestibular lesions
	direction of nystagmus varies with the direction of gaze	brainstem pathology
	upbeat nystagmus	lesions at or around the superior colliculi
	downbeat nystagmus	lesions at or around the foramen magnum
rotatory	specific to one head position, and fatigues with repeated testing	unilateral labyrinthine pathology
rotatory or mixed		brainstem pathology

Fig. 17.6 Causes of nystagmus.

Clinical syndromes of the trigeminal nerve	
Site of lesion	**Pattern of sensory loss**
supranuclear	contralateral discriminative sensory loss in lesions of the primary sensory cortex
	contralateral loss of all modalities in lesions of the internal capsule
upper pons	ipsilateral loss of light touch*, with preserved pain and temperature sensation
lower pons, medulla, upper cervical cord (lesion above C2)	contralateral loss of pain and temperature sensation in an "onion skin" distribution; preserved light touch*
cerebellopontine angle	ipsilateral loss of all modalities
cavernous sinus	ipsilateral loss of all modalities in the V_1 and occasionally V_2 distribution
trigeminal root, ganglion, and peripheral branches of the nerve	loss of all sensory modalities in the V_{1-3} distributions; there may be a more selective distribution of loss with lesions of the peripheral nerve

Fig. 17.7 Clinical syndromes of the trigeminal nerve.

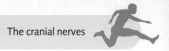

Facial (seventh) nerve
Motor

Inspect the patient's face, looking for asymmetry of the nasolabial folds and the position of the two angles of the mouth. Assess the movements of the upper part of the face by asking the patient to:

* Elevate his or her eyebrows.
* Close his or her eyes tightly and resist your attempt to open them. Look for Bell's phenomenon—this is a reflex upward deviation of the eyes in response to forced closure of the eyelids.

Movements of the lower part of the face are assessed by asking the patient to:

* Blow out his or her cheeks with air.
* Purse his or her lips tightly together and resist your attempt to open them.
* Show his or her teeth.
* Whistle.
* Smile (observe any facial asymmetry).

If you detect any weakness or asymmetry, decide if the weakness is confined to the lower part of the face (upper motor neuron lesion) or both the upper and the lower parts of the face (lower motor neuron lesion) (Fig. 17.8). Do not miss bilateral facial weakness. In this case, the face appears to sag, with lack of facial expression.

Hyperacusis (undue sensitivity to noise) is suggestive of a lesion proximal to the nerve to the stapedius.

Sensory
Taste

Taste is examined by applying a solution of salt, sweet (sugar), or sour (vinegar) to the anterior two-thirds of the tongue and comparing the response on the two sides. The mouth should be rinsed with water between testing. Lesions of the chorda tympani will cause loss of taste.

Vestibulocochlear (eighth) nerve
Hearing

Clinical bedside assessment of hearing is not sensitive and can detect only gross hearing loss. Audiometry is usually required for detailed assessment.

Assess each ear separately while masking the hearing in the other ear by occluding the external meatus with your index finger. Test the patient's hearing sensitivity by whispering numbers into his or her ear and asking him or her to repeat them.

Determine if the hearing loss is conductive or sensorineural by performing Rinne's and Weber's tests (see Chapter 8).

Vestibular function

There are no satisfactory bedside tests for vestibular function. Examination of the patient's gait and eye movements for nystagmus may be helpful; the findings in a patient who has vestibular dysfunction are summarized in Fig. 9.1. The use of caloric testing and the Hallpike maneuver for patients presenting with positional vertigo is discussed on pp. 52 and 54.

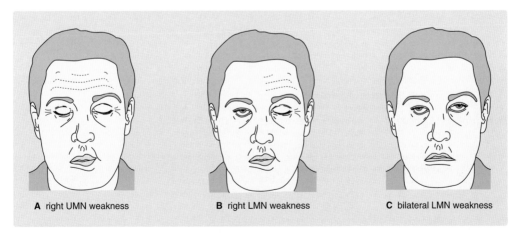

A right UMN weakness   **B** right LMN weakness   **C** bilateral LMN weakness

Fig. 17.8 Facial weakness. The patient is asked to close the eyes and purse the lips. Note the defective eye closure and Bell's phenomenon in (B) and (C). (LMN, lower motor neuron; UMN, upper motor neuron.)

A patient suspected of having vestibular dysfunction should have formal vestibular testing.

Glossopharyngeal (ninth) and vagus (tenth) nerves
Motor
Check the patient's speech (hoarse and quiet) and quality of cough to assess for dysphonia; nasal intonation of speech arises from palatal weakness.

Palatal movement can be assessed by:
- Asking the patient to say "ah" (voluntary activity).
- Touching the posterior pharyngeal wall with the end of a cotton swab on both sides (the gag reflex).

The afferent pathway of the gag reflex (ninth cranial nerve) can be assessed by asking the patient whether sensation is comparable on both sides. The efferent pathway (tenth cranial nerve) can be assessed by observing the normal response of a symmetrical rise of the soft palate and movement of the pharyngeal muscles; characteristically a gagging sound is made.

Supranuclear (upper motor neuron) innervation of the palatal and pharyngeal muscles is bilateral; therefore, unilateral lesions will not cause significant dysfunction. In patients who have bilateral upper motor neuron lesions, the palate cannot be elevated voluntarily but moves normally when testing the gag reflex ("pseudobulbar palsy").

If the voluntary and reflex movements are bilaterally impaired ("bulbar palsy") or the palate does not elevate on one side, the lesion involves the lower motor neuron. In unilateral lower motor neuron lesions the palate lies slightly lower on the affected side and deviates toward the unaffected side.

Minor and inconsistent deviations of the uvula should be ignored.

Sensory
The posterior pharyngeal wall is innervated by the glossopharyngeal (ninth cranial) nerve, and sensation is tested by a cotton swab as described above.

Accessory (eleventh) nerve
The spinal part of the accessory nerve is a purely motor nerve that arises from the upper five segments of the cervical cord. It supplies the trapezius and sternocleidomastoid muscles. Wasting of the muscles should be noted on inspection.

The strength of the sternocleidomastoid muscles is assessed by asking the patient to turn his or her head to each side against the resistance of the examiner's hand.

The strength of the trapezius muscles is assessed by asking the patient to shrug his or her shoulders upward against resistance. The bulk of the muscles is noted on palation.

Hypoglossal (twelfth) nerve
The hypoglossal nerve is a purely motor nerve that supplies the muscles of the tongue. Inspect the tongue as it lies in the floor of the mouth for evidence of wasting (which may be unilateral or bilateral), fasciculations (shivering movements at the tongue surface) or other involuntary movements.

Ask the patient to protrude the tongue. Abnormalities caused by upper and lower motor neuron lesions are summarized in Fig. 17.9.

Clinical patterns of tongue weakness		
lower motor neuron lesions	unilateral	atrophy and fasciculations ipsilateral to the side of the lesion; deviation of the tongue towards the affected side
	bilateral	bilateral atrophy and fasciculations (see bulbar palsy, p. 55)
upper motor neuron lesions	unilateral	slight deviation of the tongue away from the side of the lesion
	bilateral	tongue has limited protrusion and appears contracted (see pseudobulbar palsy, p. 55)

Fig. 17.9 Clinical patterns of tongue weakness.

The motor system

The examination should start by simply observing the patient; important information may have already been obtained through observing the patient during history taking.

Inspection
The following features should be noted on inspection:

- Posture—look for the characteristic posturing of a patient with a hemiparesis (see Fig. 13.2). Ask the patient to hold out both arms in front of the body with eyes closed; look for any drift of the arm downward from the horizontal. This provides a quick assessment of pyramidal, proprioceptive, and cerebellar function, all of which are required to maintain posture.
- Muscle wasting—look for the degree and distribution of muscle wasting. This is usually characteristic of lower motor neuron disorders (i.e., anterior horn cell, nerve root, plexus or peripheral nerve disorders).
- Fasciculations—these are seen as a rippling or twitching of the muscle at rest and are also a feature of lower motor neuron disorders.
- Involuntary movements (e.g., a resting tremor may be evident in patients who have Parkinson's disease). (See Chapter 12.)

Tone
Tone refers to the activity of the stretch reflexes assessed by the degree of resistance that occurs on stretching a muscle at different speeds.

Some patients have difficulty relaxing during an examination, which can artificially increase stiffness in their limbs. Relaxation can be achieved by asking the patient to loosen up their limbs so that they are limp.

Arms
To examine tone in the arms, relax the patient. Take the patient's arm and slowly flex and extend the elbow, then hold his or her hand, with the elbow flexed, and pronate and supinate the forearm. If tone is increased, you may feel a "supinator catch," an interruption of the smooth movement on supination.

A "cog-wheel" rigidity may be noted in patients who have Parkinson's disease; this may be enhanced by asking the patient to move the other arm up and down.

Legs
There are several ways to examine tone in the legs:

- Rock each leg from side to side on the bed, holding it at the knee. Normally, the foot lags behind the leg. If tone is increased, the foot and leg move stiffly together. If tone is decreased, the foot moves limply from side to side with each movement.
- Passively flex and extend the knee at varying speeds, supporting both the upper leg and the foot.
- With the patient's legs extended on the exam table, place your hand under the patient's knee and quickly lift the knee about 6 inches; normally, the foot will stay on the bed. If tone is increased, it may jump up with the lower leg; if tone is decreased the limb will feel lax and slightly heavier than normal.

"Clonus" describes the rhythmic, unidirectional contractions evoked by a sudden passive stretch of a muscle, elicited most easily at the ankle. A few beats may be normal, but "sustained clonus" is characteristic of an upper motor neuron lesion.

Power
Power is tested in each of the main muscle groups and graded against resistance applied by the examiner. Power in each muscle is given a grade defined by the Medical Research Council (MRC) scale (Fig. 17.10).

The MRC scale	
Grade	Response
0	no movement
1	flicker of muscle when patient tries to move
2	moves, but not against gravity
3	moves against gravity but not against resistance
4	moves against resistance but not to full strength
5	full strength (you cannot overcome the movement)

Fig. 17.10 The MRC scale for assessment of muscle power.

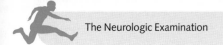
The scheme in Fig. 17.11 allows testing of the main muscle groups of the arms. The scheme in Fig. 17.12 allows testing of the main muscle groups of the legs.

Fig. 17.13 summarizes the different findings depending on the site of the pathology in patients who present with limb weakness.

> Increased tone may be due to an upper motor neuron or extrapyramidal disorder. In patients who have increased tone due to an upper motor neuron lesion there will be spasticity—look for a supinator catch, clasp-knife phenomenon and clonus, brisk reflexes, and extensor plantar responses. In patients who have increased tone due to an extrapyramidal disorder there is characteristic rigidity ("lead-pipe" rigidity) with "cog-wheeling" if there is a superimposed tremor. The reflexes are usually normal and plantar responses flexor.

Reflexes

Tendon reflexes are most easily determined by briskly stretching the tendon with a reflex hammer, held near the end and briskly tapped either onto the tendon directly or onto a finger placed over the tendon (biceps and brachioradialis). The tendon reflexes shown in Fig. 17.14A should be examined. These may be:

- Normal.
- Increased.
- Decreased.
- Absent.

If absent, this should be confirmed by reinforcement (Fig. 17.14C). Abdominal reflexes can be tested as shown in Fig. 17.14D. The plantar response is elicited by scratching the sole of the foot (Fig. 17.14E).

Tendon reflexes are conventionally annotated as shown in Fig. 17.15.

Coordination

Whether a patient can perform smooth and accurate movements is dependent on power and coordination. Weakness may give rise to apparent clumsiness, which may be misinterpreted as incoordination.

Cerebellar dysfunction gives rise to incoordination. This can be assessed as outlined below.

Gait

A wide-based, sometimes lurching gait is seen in cerebellar disease. Unsteadiness is made more obvious if the patient is asked to walk heel-to-toe in a straight line.

Arms

Cerebellar dysfunction can be assessed as follows:

- The finger–nose test—ask the patient to touch your finger, held about 20 inches in front of the patient, with his or her index finger and then to touch his or her nose, then move back and forth between your finger and the patient's nose. In patients who have a cerebellar lesion, on placing the index finger on the examiner's finger there may be a coarse oscillating tremor that is more marked as the finger approaches the examiner's finger (intention tremor). There is inability to carry out smooth and accurate movements. The latter are jerky with overshooting (past-pointing) of the target, i.e., the examiner's finger. This is known as dysmetria.
- Dysdiadokokinesis—the inability to carry out rapid alternating movements with regularity. This can be tested by asking the patient to alternately pronate and supinate his or her arm and correspondingly tap the palm and then dorsum of his or her hand on the examiner's palm. The speed of movement decreases and amplitude of movements increases.
- The "rebound phenomenon"—if the wrists are gently tapped when the arms are outstretched, the arm is displaced through a greater range of movement than normal due to failure of fixation of the arm at the shoulder by hypotonic muscles.

Legs

The heel–knee–shin test—ask the patient to place one heel on the other knee and slowly slide the heel down the lower leg, then to lift the leg up again and repeat the test. Rapid tapping movement of the feet

Fig. 17.11 Testing muscle groups of the upper limb. The green arrow indicates the direction of movement of the patient, and the black arrow the direction of movement of the examiner. Each muscle group should be given a grade as defined by the MRC scale (see Fig. 17.10).

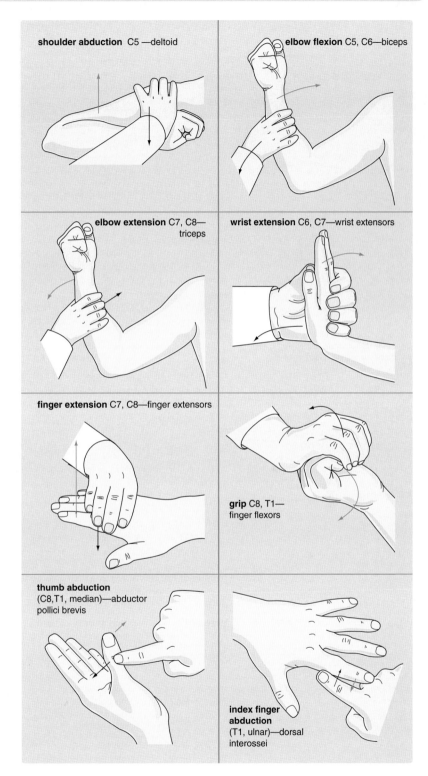

shoulder abduction C5 —deltoid

elbow flexion C5, C6—biceps

elbow extension C7, C8— triceps

wrist extension C6, C7—wrist extensors

finger extension C7, C8—finger extensors

grip C8, T1— finger flexors

thumb abduction (C8,T1, median)—abductor pollici brevis

index finger abduction (T1, ulnar)—dorsal interossei

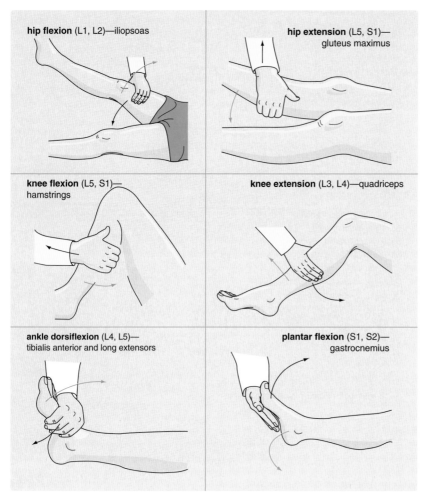

hip flexion (L1, L2)—iliopsoas

hip extension (L5, S1)—
gluteus maximus

knee flexion (L5, S1)—
hamstrings

knee extension (L3, L4)—quadriceps

ankle dorsiflexion (L4, L5)—
tibialis anterior and long extensors

plantar flexion (S1, S2)—
gastrocnemius

Fig. 17.12 Testing muscle groups of the lower limb. The red arrow indicates the direction of movement of the patient and the black arrow the direction of movement of the examiner. Each muscle group should be given a grade as defined by the MRC scale (see Fig. 17.10).

Clinical features of patterns presenting with limb weakness					
Site of lesion	Wasting	Tone	Pattern of weakness	Reflexes	Plantar response
upper motor neuron	none	increased	"pyramidal" pattern weakness	increased	extensor
lower motor neuron	present	decreased	individual or groups of muscles	decreased	flexor
neuromuscular junction	uncommon	usually normal, may be decreased	bilateral and predominantly of the proximal limb girdle (fatiguable)	usually normal	flexor
muscle	sometimes	decreased in proportion to wasting	bilateral and predominantly of the proximal limb girdle	decreased in proportion to wasting	flexor

Fig. 17.13 Variation in examination findings with site of pathology. Not every patient will have every feature, and occasionally patients may diverge from these features, but this remains a useful guide.

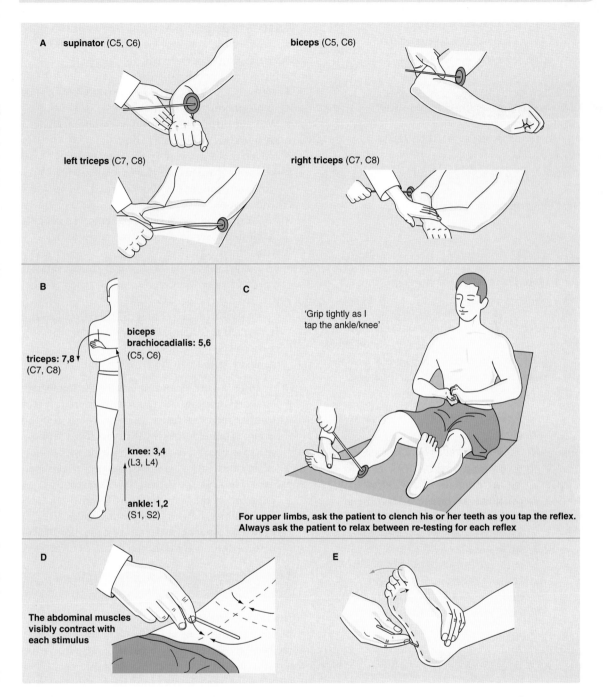

Fig. 17.14 Eliciting reflexes. (A) Upper limb tendon reflexes. (B) A simple way to remember root values of reflexes. (C) Testing ankle jerk reinforcement. (D) Abdominal reflexes: test in the four quadrants shown. (E) Plantar reflex. The normal response is a downgoing great toe. In an upper motor neuron lesion, the great toe dorsiflexes and the other toes fan out (the Babinski response).

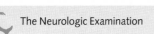

Annotation of tendon reflexes	
	Grading
absent	0
present with reinforcement only (decreased)	1
normal	2
brisk	3
very brisk, with associated clonus	4

Fig. 17.15 Annotation of tendon reflexes.

is impaired. These tests should be performed on each side in turn.

Abnormality of these movements tested above in a patient who has a cerebellar lesion is termed ataxia, and may be associated with other signs of cerebellar disease such as nystagmus and dysarthria (see Chapter 11).

> Early stages of an upper motor neuron or extrapyramidal disorder may be picked up by noting impairment of fine finger movements: ask the patient to pretend to play a piano and to touch each of his or her fingers in turn with the thumb of the same hand.

Gait

In normal gait, the erect moving body is supported by one leg at a time while the other swings forward in preparation for the next support move. Only one foot will be on the floor at any time, although both the heel of the front foot and the toes of the back foot will be on the ground momentarily when the body weight is transferred from one leg to the other. Normal gait requires input from the motor, sensory, cerebellar, and vestibular systems.

Assessment

Watch the patient walk along a stretch of corridor and observe the characteristics of the gait.

Note whether the patient:
- Walks unaided—if not, does the patient walk with a cane or crutches.
- Walks in a straight line—patients who are ataxic are unsteady and unable to do so.
- Has normal arm swing—arm swing may be reduced in patients who have a parkinsonian syndrome; this may be more marked on one side than the other.
- Can turn around with ease—patients who have a parkinsonian syndrome or ataxia perform this with difficulty.
- Can walk heel-to-toe—this will exacerbate ataxia if present; note whether the patient tends to veer towards a particular side.
- Can stand on his or her toes (S1) and then heels (L5—such as patients with a common peroneal nerve palsy)—patients with a spastic or hemiparetic gait may find this difficult.

Other steps in gait assessment include the following:
- Romberg's test—ask the patient to stand with feet together and eyes closed. The test is positive if the patient is more unsteady with eyes closed than with eyes open; this occurs in patients with a sensory ataxia who have impaired proprioception.
- Stress gait—ask the patient to walk on the "outsides" of the feet. With corticospinal tract abnormalities, patients will posture hands.
- If gait appears abnormal, classify it into one of the patterns described in Chapter 15.

The sensory system

Patients use various terms to describe sensory disturbance, including numbness, tingling, "pins and needles," and burning. Medical terms include paresthesia (tingling), dysesthesia (unpleasant awareness of touch or pressure), hyperesthesia (exaggeration of any sensation), and hyperalgesia (exaggerated perception of painful stimuli).

Test each sensation in turn, starting with the fingers and toes and work proximally. Ask the patient to indicate "yes" when he or she perceives each sensation and compare the right and left sides. Explain what you are going to do first and ensure that the patient's eyes are closed during the examination.

Sensory testing

Do not spend hours doing sensory testing—you will exhaust the patient and yourself. Be sensible, and tailor your examination to the patient's complaint.

If the patient complains of loss or impairment of sensation, start sensory testing in the abnormal area and move out from there.

Patterns of sensory impairmant are discussed in Chapter 14.

Pin prick

Use a sensory-testing or safety pin, not a hypodermic needle. This tests pain sensation. The patient should be able to differentiate the sharp and blunt ends of the pin. Ask the patient whether the sensation feels sharp or blunt.

Temperature

A cold object such as the flat surface of a nonvibrating tuning fork can be used to test perception of cold temperature.

Light touch

A wisp of cotton is used to test light touch. Remember that "tickle" is carried by spinothalamic fibers.

Joint-position sense

Move the distal interphalangeal (DIP) joint of the index finger/big toe up or down, holding the sides of the digit. Ask the patient to indicate the direction in which the digit is being moved. If perception of joint position is abnormal, gradually move proximally (e.g., wrist, elbow, shoulder).

Vibration

Use a 128-Hz tuning fork. Set it vibrating and place it on the patient's chin. Ask the patient whether he or she can feel this vibrating. If so, place the tuning fork on the DIP joint of the finger/big toe and ask the patient whether he or she can feel it vibrating here. If the patient cannot feel it move proximally, e.g. lateral malleoli, tibial tuberosity, iliac crest, sternum. You may find a sensory level.

Vibration sense is often lost early in peripheral neuropathies.

General examination

Always conclude with examination of the other systems. In particular take note of the cardiovascular examination.

The blood pressure should be recorded while the patient lies supine and again after standing for a couple of minutes to check for postural hypotension. The systolic blood pressure usually rises a little; a fall of more than 20 mmHg is abnormal.

The blood pressure of patients who have suspected cerebrovascular insufficiency should be tested in both arms.

Sample neurology history and physical (H&P)

Details

Name: *Joanna Kopinski*
Date: *2/19/05*
Age: *29*
Sex: *Female*
Occupation: *Secretary*
Handedness: *Right-handed*

Admitted from the outpatient clinic following urgent PCP referral.

CC (chief complaint)
Two-week history of difficulty walking.

HPI (history of presenting illness)
Two-week history of progressive difficulty in walking.
Initially: tendency to trip over on left leg—two occasions of catching her left foot on the curb and falling.
Currently: she is finding it difficult to maneuver both legs and catches both feet when climbing the curb or stairs.
There is no pain. Her walking has gradually deteriorated.
No visual symptoms currently (reduction in visual acuity, central field defect, double vision).
No problems with speech and swallowing.
No symptoms in her arms.

She has also developed mild urgency and frequency of urination over the previous week. This is not associated with burning or pain.

At the age of 20, she had an episode of pain and visual vrination in the left eye. This settled after 6 weeks. No treatment was given. She was told this was due to "neuritis."

Medications
Oral contraceptive pill.

PMH (past medical history)
1983: Appendicectomy.
1989: Visual loss—"neuritis" for 6 weeks.

FH (family history)
No significant FH/no FH of neurologic diseases.
Father, mother, and siblings alive and well.

SH (social history)

Works as a secretary.

Smokes 20 cigarettes per day (since aged 18).

Alcohol—10 drinks per week.

Occasionally smokes marijuana; no other illicit drugs.

Sexual history: lives with boyfriend of 8 years; four previous sexual partners.

Travel history: recent travel to Europe only.

Pets: none.

ROS (review of systems)

General: Marked fatigue recently

CVS: No chest pain/palpitations/orthopnea/paroxysmal nocturnal dyspnea (PND)

RS: No cough/sputum/wheeze

GI: Appetite and weight stable

No change in bowel habit

GUS: Recent urgency and frequency

No burning/pain

NS: As above

Skin: No rash/pruritis/bruising

Others: Negative

P/E (physical examination)

General: Anxious woman, no apparent distress

Vitals: BP 130/70, P 80 regular, weight 125 lbs

Cardiac: Heart sounds—normal, peripheral pulses—all present, no bruits

Lungs: Clear to A&P

Abdomen: Soft/nontender

No liver/spleen/kidneys palpable

Neuro

MS: A, O x 3, fluent, nl att & conc, regis 3/3, recall 3/3 at 5 mins

Higher functions intact

Cranial nerves:

II VA 20/20 OD, 20/100 OS

Ishihara plates (color vision): R 17/17; L 3/17

Left relative afferent pupillary defect

Desaturation to red pin centrally in L eye, otherwise normal visual fields

Fundi: pale disc on L

III/IV/VI Horizontal nystagmus on lateral gaze

V–XII: intact

Motor exam

Upper limbs: Tone: Normal

Power: 5/5 all muscle groups—drift

Lower limbs: Tone: Increased tone bilaterally (L > R)

Power:	R	L
Hip flexion	$4^+/5$	$4^-/5$
Hip extension	5/5	5/5
Knee flexion	4/5	3/5
Knee extension	5/5	5/5
Ankle dorsiflexion	$4^-/5$	3/5
Ankle plantarflexion	5/5	5/5

Coordination: Intention tremor on finger–nose testing bilaterally (L>R)

Difficult to test heel-shin reliably with the degree of weakness

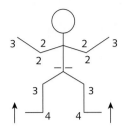

Sensation: Normal light touch (LT), pinprick (PP), joint-position sense (JPS), and vibration (vib) in both upper and lower limbs

Gait: Spastic gait—L worse than R (stiff legs—extended legs circumduct to try and avoid scuffing the toes)

Assessment/Plan:

A 29-year-old woman, with a previous history of temporary visual loss in the left eye, presents with a 2-week history of progressive difficulty in walking. There is unilateral optic atrophy, with nystagmus in both eyes, no evidence of an INO, and mild incoordination in the arms. There is an asymmetrical spastic paraparesis with bladder involvement. Differential diagnosis is multiple sclerosis, transverse myelitis, disc disease, spinal cord tumor, spinal cord AVM, Lyme disease, metastatic tumor.

Problem list

1. *Confirm diagnosis of multiple sclerosis/rule out spinal cord compression—magnetic resonance imaging (brain/spinal cord); lumbar puncture (?positive oligoclonal bands); visual evoked potentials.*
2. *Treatment—intravenous methylprednisolone [check for urinary tract infection (UTI) and treat if present]; physical therapy.*
3. *Social/psychological factors—discussion about diagnosis, prognosis, and any plans and adaptations that may be required (short or long term).*
4. *Follow-up—for further discussion and support, to catch signs of relapse early, to prevent complications of the disease (UTI, pressure sores, etc.) and to assess suitability for β-interferon.*

19. Further Investigations

Routine investigations

You should be aware of simple tests of neurologic relevance. In this section, five areas of investigation are presented:

- Hematology (Fig. 19.1).
- Biochemistry (Fig. 19.2).
- Immunology (Fig. 19.3).
- Microbiology (Fig. 19.4).
- Cerebrospinal fluid findings.

For each test, normal ranges are given, with neurologic differential diagnoses for high and low values.

Neurophysiologic investigations

Electroencephalography (EEG)

EEG measures electrical potentials generated by the neurons lying underneath an electrode on the scalp, and compares these with recordings from either a reference electrode or a neighboring electrode. The normal trace is symmetrical; therefore, asymmetries as well as specific abnormalities may indicate an underlying disorder.

Before accurate brain imaging was possible, EEG was used to detect focal lesions. These are now more commonly picked up with computed tomography (CT) or magnetic resonance (MR) imaging, but EEG remains useful for detecting underlying abnormalities of cerebral function, and especially for:

- Epilepsy (see below).
- Diagnosis of encephalitis (especially herpes simplex infection).
- Coma.
- Aid to diagnosis of Creutzfeldt–Jakob disease.
- Diagnosis of subacute sclerosing panencephalitis.

The main role of EEG is in the assessment of epilepsy. It can help in the following ways:

- Diagnosis (although this is made primarily on the clinical history, and the EEG may be normal in patients who have clearly had seizures): an increased yield of abnormalities may be obtained if recording is made under conditions of sleep deprivation, with hyperventilation, and with photic stimulation.
- Classification of seizure type, which may optimize therapy.
- Assessment for surgical intervention.
- Diagnosis of pseudoseizures (especially with simultaneous video recording—telemetry).

Intracranial EEG monitoring refers to prolonged recording from electrodes inserted directly into the brain, undertaken before surgery to remove an epileptic focus.

Different normal rhythms are characteristically found over different regions of the brain (Fig. 19.5). Other than these rhythmic activities, other abnormal activity may be generated in certain conditions (Figs. 19.6 and 19.7).

Electromyography (EMG) and nerve conduction studies (NCS)

EMG and NCS, usually performed together, examine the integrity of muscle, peripheral nerve, and lower motor neurons. They are useful in:

- Determining the cause of weakness (e.g., neuropathy, myopathy, anterior horn cell disease).
- Determining the distribution of the abnormality (e.g., generalized or focal).
- Suggesting the type of myopathy (e.g., dystrophy or myositis) or neuropathy (e.g., axonal or demyelinating; motor, sensory, or sensorimotor).
- Diagnosing Myasthenia Gravis.
- Assessing baseline deficits before surgery (e.g., carpal tunnel syndrome).
- Objectively assessing the response to medical therapies, especially new treatments in trials (e.g., human immunoglobulin in Guillain Barré syndrome).

EMG

EMG involves the insertion of a needle electrode into muscle.

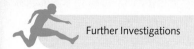

Hemotology			
Test	Normal range	Abnormality	Possible interpretation
complete blood count (CBC)			
hemoglobin (Hb)	13.5–18.0g/dL male; 11.5–16.0g/dL female	low; anemia	may cause nonspecific neurologic symptoms (e.g., dizziness, weakness, fainting); may suggest an underlying chronic illness, associated with restless legs syndrome
		high; polycythaemia	predisposes to stroke and chorea
mean cell volume (MCV)	76–96fL	high; macrocytic anemia	vitamin B_{12} deficiency (peripheral neuropathy, SCDC, dementia)
		low; microcytic anemia	may indicate an underlying chronic illness; associated with idiopathic intracranial hypertension
white cell count (WBC)			
neutrophils	$2–7.5 \times 10^9$/L	high; neutrophilia	meningitis or other infection
		low; neutropenia	leukemia or lymphoma (infiltrative disease, space-occupying lesions, peripheral neuropathy) multiple myeloma (neuropathy, vertebral collapse, hyperviscosity syndrome)
lymphocytes	$1.5–3.5 \times 10^9$/L	high; lymphocytosis	viral infection (transverse myelitis, Guillain–Barré syndrome)
		low; lymphopenia	leukemia or lymphoma, as above
eosinophils	$0.04–0.44 \times 10^9$/L	high; eosinophilia	hypereosinophilic syndrome (rare)
platelet count	$150–400 \times 10^9$/L	high; thrombocythemia	predisposes to stroke
		low; thrombocytopenia	bleeding
erythrocyte sedimentation rate (ESR)	<20mm/h	high	vasculitis (e.g. PAN, SLE, giant-cell arteritis) may cause cerebral, cranial, and peripheral nerve infarcts, confusion and seizures)
coagulation tests			
activated partial thromboplastin time (APT or PTTK)	35–45s	high	SLE; antiphospholipid syndrome
protein C, protein S	varies with laboratory	low; deficiency	inherited predisposition to thrombosis (arterial and venous)
factor 5 Leiden	varies with laboratory	present	mutation causes a single amino acid substitution in factor 5, which results in activated protein C resistance and predisposition to thrombosis (arterial and venous)
vitamin B_{12}	>150 ng/L	low; deficiency	peripheral neuropathy, SCDC, confusion/dementia
folate	4–18 µg/L	low; deficiency	peripheral neuropathy, dementia

Fig. 19.1 Possible consequences of abnormalities in blood or serum levels of hematologic indices. Individual laboratories may have different normal ranges. (APT, activated thromboplastin; PAN, polyarteritis nodosa; PTTK, partial thromboplastin time; SCDC, subacute combined degeneration of the cord; SLE, systemic lupus erythematosus.)

Biochemistry			
Test	**Normal range**	**Abnormality**	**Interpretation**
electrolytes			
sodium	135–145 mmol/L	high; hypernatremia low; hyponatremia	both may cause weakness, confusion, and seizures
potassium	3.5–5.5 mmol/L	high; hyperkalemia low; hypokalemia	hyper- or hypokalemic periodic paralysis
urea	2.5–6.7 mmol/L	high; renal failure	confusion, peripheral neuropathy
creatinine	<120 mmol/L	high; renal failure	confusion, peripheral neuropathy
glucose (fasting)	4–6 mmol/L	high; diabetes low; hypoglycemia	neuropathy, coma confusion, coma, focal signs
calcium	2.2–2.6 mmol/L	high; hypercalcemia low; hypocalcemia	cancer tetany, seizures
liver function tests (LFTs) bilirubin and liver enzymes	bilirubin range: 3–17 mmol/L enzyme levels vary between laboratories	high	liver disease: confusion, tremor, neuropathy
creatine kinase (CK)	24–195 U/L	high	muscle disease: myositis, muscular dystrophy
thyroid function tests thyroid-stimulating hormone (TSH)	0.5–5.0 mU/L	low TSH; thyrotoxisis high TSH; hypothyroidism	tremor, confusion, hyperreflexia apathy, confusion, hyporeflexia, neuropathy, dementia
thyroxine (T_4)	10–24 pmol/L	low: hypothyroidism high: thyrotoxicosis	apathy, confusion, hyporeflexia, neuropathy, dementia tremor, confusion, hyperreflexia

Fig. 19.2 Possible consequences of abnormalities in blood or serum levels of biochemical indices. Individual laboratories may have different normal ranges.

Normal muscle at rest is electrically silent (apart from actually during needle insertion—insertional activity), unless the needle is placed in the region of a motor end-plate (when miniature end-plate potentials are recorded).

In abnormal muscles, either due to primary muscle disease or to denervation of the muscle, spontaneous activity may be seen at rest. The most common types of spontaneous activity include fibrillation potentials, positive sharp waves and fasciculations.

Fibrillations potentials and positive sharp waves are due to spontaneous contractions of individual muscle fibers, probably due to abnormal rhythmic fluctuations of membrane potential. They cannot be seen through the skin. They are most commonly seen in denervation but may be found in some muscle diseases especially inflammatory muscle disease (e.g., polymyositis).

Fasciculation potentials are much larger than fibrillations and represent the contractions of groups of muscle fibers supplied by a motor unit. They occur following denervation. They may be seen as a ripple through the skin. They are common in motor neuron disease. Fasciculations may occur as normal phenomenon, especially after excess caffeine or in thyrotoxicosis. However, in these situations the firing rate is far more rapid than in diseases caused by denervation.

During voluntary movement, individual motor unit potentials (MUPs; the activity of a single anterior horn cell) can be seen. Common abnormalities of EMG are shown in Fig. 19.8.

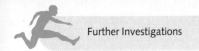

Immunology	
Test	**Associated disorder**
antinuclear factor (ANA)	systemic lupus erythematosus (SLE): seizures, confusion, neuropathy, aseptic meningitis, Sjögren's syndrome: dry eyes, neuropathies, mixed connective tissue disease (MCTD)
anti-double-stranded DNA (dsDNA) antibodies	SLE
rheumatoid factor	rheumatoid arthritis: cervical spine subluxation, neuropathies, vasculitis
anti-Ro (SSA), anti-La (SSB) antibodies	Sjögren's syndrome
antiphospholipid antibodies (e.g. anticardiolipin)	antiphospholipid syndrome
anti-ribonucleoprotein (RNP) antibodies	MCTD; myositis, trigeminal nerve palsies
Jo-1 antibodies	polymyositis
antineutrophil cytoplasmic antibodies (ANCA)	pANCA (peripheral): polyarteritis nodosa cANCA (classical): Wegener's granulomatosis
anti-acetylcholine receptor (AChR) antibodies/ antimuscle-specific receptor	myasthenia gravis tyrosine kinase (Mu Sk) antibodies
anti-GM1 antibodies	multifocal motor neuropathy, Gullain–Barré syndrome
anti-GAD antibodies	stiff-man syndrome

Fig. 19.3 Immunology: autoantibodies and their associated syndromes.

Microbiology	
Test	**Associated disorder**
bacterial microscopy and culture (including blood, CSF, urine, stool, sputum and wounds)	bacterial infections can cause a wide range of conditions—septicemia, meningitis, pneumonia, urinary tract infections, cerebral abscess etc. or are implicated in their pathogenesis, e.g., Guillain Barré syndrome (*Campylobacterpylori*)
	do not forget atypical infections caused by Listeria, Mycoplasma, Legionella etc.; diagnosis of TB requires special stains (Ziehl–Neelsen) and culture media (Lowenstein–Jensen)
viral serology and culture (blood, CSF)	viruses can cause a wide range of neurological infections, e.g., meningitis, encephalitis, shingles (herpes zoster)
VDRL (venereal disease reference laboratory) (blood)	primary syphilis (false positives—pregnancy, systemic lupus erythematosus, malaria)
TPA (*Treponema pallidum* hemagglutination assay) (blood)	syphilis, false positives—as VDRL and other treponemal infections (yaws, pinto)
Borrelia serology (blood, CSF)	Lyme disease (see Chapter 33)
HIV (blood)	AIDS (see Chapter 33)
HTLV-1 (blood)	myelopathy

Fig. 19.4 Microbiology: investigations that should be carried out if infections are implicated as the cause of neurologic disease.

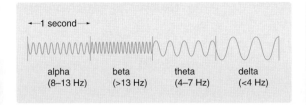

Fig. 19.5 Normal electroencephalographic rhythms.

Some abnormal EEG activities	
Activity	**Interpretation**
generalized slowing	metabolic encephalopathy, drug overdose, encephalitis
focal slowing	underlying white matter structural lesion
focal or generalized spikes, or spike and slow-wave activity	epilepsy
three-per-second (3/s), bilateral, symmetrical spike-and-wave activity (Fig. 19.7)	typical absence seizures and other "primary generalized epilepsy" syndromes
periodic complexes (generalized sharp waves every 0.5–2.0 seconds)	CJD

Fig. 19.6 Some abnormal electroencephalographic activities.

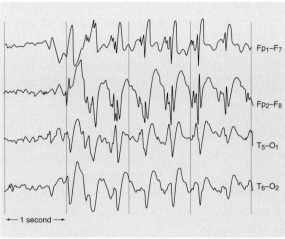

Fig. 19.7 Three-per-second (3/s) spike-and-wave activity, characteristic of typical absence seizure.

Nerve conduction studies (NCS)

NCS involve stimulating a nerve with an electrical impulse via a surface electrode and recording further along the nerve (sensory studies) or recording the muscle action potential (motor studies).

The amplitude of the response, the latency to the beginning of the response and the conduction velocity are measured. As a general rule, a reduction in conduction velocity suggests demyelination, whereas reduction in amplitude suggest axonal loss (see Fig. 19.8).

Evoked potentials (EPs)

These use EEG electrodes to record responses centrally to peripheral stimuli—visual, auditory, and electrical stimuli from sensory nerves respectively.

- Visual EPs (VEPs)—these are delayed in patients who have had an episode of optic neuritis (whether or not this resulted in temporary loss of sight) and this is therefore a useful test to help confirm a diagnosis of multiple sclerosis.
- Brainstem auditory EPs (BAEPs).
- Somatosensory EPs (SSEPs).

Magnetic brain stimulation

This test applies a magnetic pulse over the motor cortex and records the response in a muscle in the arm or leg, thereby assessing central motor conduction time.

Imaging of the nervous system

Plain radiography
Skull radiography

Skull radiography has a limited role in current neurologic practice. The main indication is head injury when more sophisticated imaging is not immediately indicated. The standard views are:
- Lateral.
- Posteroanterior.
- Towne's view (fronto-occipital).

Spinal radiography

The standard views in spinal radiography are:
- Lateral.
- Posteroanterior.

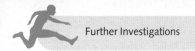

Common abnormalities found with EMG and NCS	
Abnormality	**Change in electromyographic trace**
denervation	increased insertional activity; fibrillations, positive sharp waves, and fasciculations; large amplitude, long duration, polyphasic MUPs
myopathy	small, short, polyphasic MUPs
Myasthenia Gravis	abnormal decrement of amplitude of response on repetitive stimulation using nerve conduction tests; increased "jitter" with single-fiber EMG (indicating variable neuromuscular transmission time)
Abnormality	**Change in nerve conduction**
axonal neuropathy	small action potential; normal nerve conduction velocity
demyelinating neuropathy	slow nerve conduction velocity; prolonged latency (time to travel from one point to the next); normal or slightly reduced action potential

Fig. 19.8 Common abnormalities found with electromyography (EMG) and nerve conduction studies (NCS). (MUPs, motor unit potentials.)

Computerized tomography scanning

Using an x-ray source and a series of photon detectors housed in a gantry, CT produces a series of consecutive two-dimensional axial brain digital images that show the x-ray density of the brain tissue.

The densities of different brain tissues vary according to their x-ray absorption properties, ranging from low (black: air, cerebrospinal fluid) to high (white: bone, fresh blood).

The diagnostic yield of the CT scanning is increased by injecting iodine-containing contrast agents, which enhance the distinction between the different brain tissues and outline the areas of blood–brain barrier breakdown (around tumors or infarctions).

Magnetic resonance imaging

The term nuclear magnetic resonance describes the interaction between the hydrogen protons in the different body structures and strong external magnetic fields. As the patient lies in the scanner, the naturally spinning hydrogen protons align with the strong magnetic field of the scanner. When a further external magnetic field (radiofrequency pulse) of a specific frequency is applied at a right angle, the protons "flip" out of the main external magnetic field.

As the protons "relax" back to their original position, they emit a radiofrequency signal that can be digitally analyzed and displayed as an image. This "relaxation" time has two components, known as T1 and T2, which determine the MR parameters of the different brain tissues.

The paramagnetic agent gadolinium-labelled DTPA (diethylene triamine penta-acetic acid, or pentetic acid) is used as contrast agent.

Modification of the field conditions can now produce good quality images of the cervical or the cerebral blood vessels (either arterial or venous), the technique of MR angiography.

Myelography

A water-soluble, iodine-based medium is injected in the subarachnoid space through a lumbar or a cervical approach. This outlines the spinal canal and nerve root sheaths, allowing the assessment of the spinal canal and the nerve roots. Cord compression caused by extramedullary or intramedullary lesions is identified as a compression or interruption of the column of contrast.

Postmyelographic CT scanning provides more detailed images of the nerve roots within the theca.

Imaging of the spinal cord is now performed largely by MR scanning, but myelography can be helpful in specific conditions (nerve root lesions, spinal dural arteriovenous malformation [AVM]) or in patients unable to undergo MR imaging because of claustrophobia or a cardiac pacemaker.

The advantages of MR imaging are:
- Absence of ionizing radiation.
- The ability to obtain images in coronal and sagittal as well as axial planes.
- More sensitive to the pathologic changes in the brain tissues.

The disadvantages are:
- Cannot be used for patients with pacemakers (the magnetic field interferes with their function).
- Cannot be used for patients with ferromagnetic intracranial aneurysmal clips or implants (they distort the images and could be displaced by the strong magnetic field).
- Patients who suffer from claustrophobia may be unable to tolerate the confined space within the MRI machine.

Angiography

Serial cranial radiographs are taken after the injection of an iodine-containing contrast agent into a large artery (aorta, carotid, vertebral) to allow the identification of cerebral vessels. Simultaneous digital subtraction of the surrounding soft tissues and bony structures allows the use of more-dilute contrast and a shorter procedure time, although the spatial resolution of the images will be compromised.

Venous digital subtraction angiography is possible, but the quality of the images obtained is distinctly inferior to those obtained through the arterial route.

The indications for angiography are:
- Diagnosis of extracranial atherosclerotic cerebrovascular disease (stenosis, lumen irregularities, or occlusions), when not shown by Doppler study or MR angiography.
- Diagnosis of aneurysms and arteriovenous malformation.
- Diagnosis of cerebral vasculitis and other rare angiopathies.
- Assessment of cerebral vessel anatomy and tumor blood supply before neurosurgery.
- Interventional angiography: embolization of vascular malformations.

Duplex sonography

Duplex sonography offers a combination of real-time and Doppler-flow ultrasound scanning, allowing a noninvasive assessment of extracranial arteries. It is particularly helpful as a screening test for lesions at the carotid bifurcation, which avoids the need for angiography in many patients. The quality of this technique is dependent on the experience and skill of the operator.

119

BACKGROUND INFORMATION AND MANAGEMENT PLANS

20. Dementia

Definition

Dementia is a symptom of disease, not a single disease entity.

There is global deterioration of intellect, behavior, and personality, usually progressive, secondary to diffuse involvement of the cerebral hemispheres, in an alert subject.

Memory must be impaired to make the diagnosis.

Impairment of conscious level suggests delirium, rather than dementia, and may occur as a consequence of toxic, metabolic, or infective conditions.

Epidemiology

The most common causes of dementia are Alzheimer's disease and vascular dementia, and these are predominantly diseases of the elderly.

The prevalence in persons aged between 50 and 70 years is about 1% and in those approaching 90 years reaches 50%. The annual incidence rate is 190/100,000 (with an increasing aging population, it is expected to rise).

General clinical features

The earliest feature of dementia, from most causes, is loss of memory for recent events. Subsequent symptoms include abnormal behavior, loss of intellect, mood changes, and difficulty coping with ordinary routines. Insight may be retained initially, but is then usually lost. Ultimately, there is loss of self-care, wandering, incontinence, and often paranoia.

Rate of progression depends on the underlying cause:
- Alzheimer's disease—slowly progressive over years.

- Vascular dementia—progressive but often fluctuating or stepwise with each stroke.
- Encephalitis—over days to weeks.

Note that all dementias tend to be accelerated by a change in environment, intercurrent infection, or surgical procedures.

Depression in the elderly can mimic the initial phases of dementia and is termed pseudodementia. Pseudodementia is amenable to antidepressant medications.

History and examination

It is essential to obtain a history from a relative or friend, as well as from the patient, in order to gauge the following:
- Rate of intellectual decline.
- Activities of daily living and social interaction.
- Nutritional status.
- Drug history.
- General health and relevant disorders (e.g., stroke, head injury).
- Family history of dementia.

Neurologic examination should specifically look for evidence of:
- Focal signs.
- Involuntary movements.
- Pseudobulbar signs.
- Primitive reflexes (e.g., snout, grasp, and palmomental reflexes).
- Gait disorder.

Formal assessment by a clinical psychologist is advisable, but a bedside "mini-mental" test provides

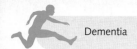
initial information about intellectual function. These tests are designed to test memory, abstract thought, judgement, and specific higher cortical functions, and should include questions similar to those listed in Fig. 17.1.

Investigations

It is important to carry out a number of investigations to exclude common and often treatable causes of dementia.

Blood tests
Routine blood tests should be performed to exclude:
- Hypothyroidism.
- Vitamin B_{12} and folate deficiency.
- Syphilis.
- Lyme disease.
- HIV infection.
- Metabolic disorders (e.g., Wilson's disease, leukodystrophy).
- Vasculitis and inflammatory diseases.

Cranial imaging
Cranial imaging can be performed using computed tomography (CT) or magnetic resonance imaging (MRI). Variable degrees of cerebral atrophy with enlarged ventricles are seen with most forms of dementia (Fig. 20.1).

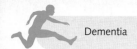

Fig. 20.1 CT scan appearances of atrophy of the brain with enlarged ventricle. This is a nonspecific finding in many causes of dementia.

It is important to exclude:
- Space-occupying lesions—especially chronic subdural hematoma in the elderly following a fall.
- Normal-pressure hydrocephalus—enlarged ventricles without cortical atrophy; presents with dementia, urinary incontinence, and gait apraxia; treated by ventriculoperitoneal shunting.

MRI and volumetric studies may show bilateral hippocampal and temporal lobe atrophy in Alzheimer's disease, and asymmetrical anterior hippocampal, amygdala, and temporal lobe atrophy in Pick's disease.

Electroencephalography (EEG)
Early slowing favors Alzheimer's disease, whereas the EEG is usually normal in Pick's disease. A completely normal EEG should raise the suspicion of depression mimicking dementia.

Periodic complexes may indicate prion disease (spongiform encephalopathy or Creutzfeldt–Jakob disease), in which the rapidly progressive course is usually an important diagnostic point.

Genetic testing
Genetic tests are rarely used for evaluation. Test for:
- Huntington mutation—Huntington's chorea.
- Amyloid precursor protein (APP) and apoliprotein E4 mutations—Alzheimer's disease.
- Prion protein gene mutation—familial Creutzfeldt–Jakob disease.

Brain biopsy
Brain biopsy is especially indicated if a treatable cause is suspected but not diagnosable by any other means (e.g., vasculitis).

Functional imaging with positron emission tomography (PET) and single photon-emitting emission computed tomography (SPECT)
PET and SPECT are techniques that measure tissue concentrations and metabolism of radioactive isotopes linked to biologically active compounds and therefore provide functional images of the brain. In Alzheimer's disease hypometabolism has been found in the posterior cingulated and neocortical association area.

Management

Treat amenable causes of dementia—some are potentially reversible (e.g., vasculitis, hydrocephalus, and pseudodementia).

In nontreatable cases, treat concurrent depression and any underlying systemic disorders.

Neuroleptic use may be required for behavioral disturbance but can exacerbate extrapyramidal features.

Management of most cases of dementia requires careful advice and counseling of the patient and family and shared care involving the family, caregivers, hospital specialist, PCP, and community psychiatric services. Long-term residential care is often required.

Primary degenerative dementia

Alzheimer's disease

Alzheimer's disease is the most common cause of dementia; scientists believe that 4.5 million Americans suffer from Alzheimer's disease. It is rarely seen in persons under the age of 45 years—the incidence increases with age.

Familial cases are occasionally seen. The loci are found on chromosome 21, associated with the gene for APP, in early-onset disease, and on chromosome 19, associated with the gene for apolipoprotein E4, in late-onset disease.

Individuals with Down's syndrome develop the full neuropathological changes of Alzheimer's disease by their fourth to fifth decade of life, probably as a consequence of the excessive APP produced by a 50% increase in gene dosage due to the extra chromosome 21.

Pathology

Alzheimer's disease is identified by the presence of senile plaques and neurofibrillary tangles in the brain.

Senile plaques consist of dystrophic neurites clustered round a core of β-amyloid protein, which is derived from a larger precursor protein, the APP.

Neurofibrillary tangles are derived from the microtubule-associated protein tau, which is in an abnormally hyperphosphorylated state.

Clinical features

Alzheimer's disease presents with classic features of a progressive dementia, often evolving over years.

It frequently results in aphasia. Pyramidal and extrapyramidal features may occur rarely.

Diagnosis

A definite diagnosis of Alzheimer' disease can be made only from pathologic findings. In practice, a typical history with progressive dementia and negative findings in routine tests will allow a diagnosis of probable Alzheimer's disease.

CT scans show nonspecific cerebral atrophy with enlarged ventricles (see Fig. 20.1).

Features found on MRI and volumetric studies add corroboration to a clinical diagnosis, as does the presence of mutations on chromosome 21 or 19 in familial cases.

PET scans are used more routinely to aid in the diagnosis.

Drug treatment

There is no cure for Alzheimer's disease. Tacrine (Cognex), donezepil (Aricept), rivastigmine (Exelon), and galantamine (Reminyl) may slow progression for patients with mild disease. Mamentine (Namenda) is approved for moderate disease. Recent studies show that the lipid-lowering statin drugs may reduce disease.

A vaccine trial was aborted after difficulties with encephalitis.

Medicines to treat sleep disorders, anxiety, and depression may control behavioral symptoms.

Prognosis

Despite advances to date, the prognosis of Alzheimer's disease is very poor, with relentless progress to death, often due to bronchopneumonia. The mean survival is 8 years from the onset of the disease.

Pick's disease

Pick's disease is a rare cause of dementia. It is accompanied by marked cerebral atrophy—greater than that seen in Alzheimer's disease—often asymmetrical and confined mainly to the frontal and/or temporal lobes.

Argyrophilic bodies, called Pick bodies, are found within the neuronal cytoplasm.

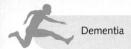

The disease is more common in women and occurs especially between the ages of 40 and 60 years.

The cause is unknown, but there is an autosomal dominant transmission in some families.

Pick's disease can be difficult to distinguish from Alzheimer's, but in the former focal frontal features are more common, the EEG is usually normal, and CT scans show prominent frontotemporal atrophy.

No specific treatment has been found, and the disease progresses to death over 2–5 years.

Vascular dementia

Large-vessel disease

Strategically localized single brain lesions may profoundly affect mental function and behavior but without causing the true syndrome of dementia.

When accompanied by other signs such as hemiparesis, diagnostic problems do not arise, but "silent" strokes can occur with behavioral features as the main characteristic.

Multi-infarct dementia

Multi-infarct dementia is the second most common cause of dementia, accounting for 10% of cases. It is caused by accumulation of defects through bilaterally localized infarcts.

It occurs mainly after the age of 50 years, with a male preponderance.

Dementia occurs in a stepwise fashion with each stroke, with episodes of focal neurologic deficit.

Often there is evidence of other vascular disease (e.g., ischemic heart disease, peripheral vascular disease) or vascular risk factors (e.g., hypertension, diabetes).

Diagnosis

The diagnosis of multi-infarct dementia is based on the history and the presence of multiple areas of infarction on CT scanning or MRI.

Note that the presence of cerebrovascular disease does not necessarily imply that the strokes have caused the dementia—concomitant Alzheimer's disease may occur.

Treatment

Treatment of multi-infarct dementia includes:
- Primary prevention for patients at risk, to prevent the onset of multiple strokes (see Chapter 31).
- Secondary prevention of atherosclerosis in established cases—control hypertension and give aspirin ± dipyridamole.

Vasculitis and microangiopathy

Vasculitis and microangiopathy are uncommon causes of dementia but should be recognized, since most cases are amenable to treatment.

They include:
- Polyarteritis nodosa.
- Primary granulomatous angiitis—isolated vasculitis of the central nervous system.
- Systemic lupus erythematosus.
- Giant-cell arteritis.
- Thrombotic microangiopathies.

Dementia as part of other degenerative diseases

Dementia occurs in a variety of neurologic disorders. In the following conditions, dementia may be prominent:
- Parkinson's disease.
- Diffuse Lewy body disease.
- Progressive supranuclear palsy.

21. Epilepsy

Definitions

Epilepsy results, physiologically speaking, from abnormal, sudden, excessive and rapid electrical discharges arising from cerebral neurons. These discharges are self-terminating but have a tendency to recur.

An *epileptic seizure* can be defined clinically as an intermittent, stereotyped disturbance of consciousness, behavior, emotion, motor function, or sensation, arising from abnormal neuronal discharges.

Epilepsy is the condition in which seizures recur, usually spontaneously.

Status epilepticus is a state of continued or recurrent seizures, with failure to regain consciousness between seizures. This is a medical emergency, with a mortality rate of 10–15%.

Prodrome refers to premonitory changes in mood or behavior—these may precede the attack by some hours.

An *aura* is the subjective sensation or phenomenon that precedes and marks the onset of the epileptic seizure—it may localize the seizure origin within the brain.

Ictus is the attack or seizure itself.

The *postictal period* is the time after the ictus during which the patient may be drowsy, confused, and disorientated.

Classification

In 1981, the International Classification of Epileptic Seizures (ICES) was proposed, and it now replaces older classifications (Fig 21.1).

Epidemiology

Ten percent of the population will suffer one seizure during their lifetime. Recurrent seizures occur in 3% of the population; 70% of these cases are well controlled with drugs and have prolonged remissions.

Epilepsy more commonly presents during childhood or adolescence but can occur at any age. Peak incidence is biphasic—early in life (age <2 years) and later in life (age >60 years).

Etiology

Epilepsy is a symptom of numerous disorders, but in 60% of patients with epilepsy, no apparent cause is found, despite full investigation.

Of the symptomatic causes in adults, vascular disease (stroke), alcohol abuse, cerebral tumors, and head injury are the most common.

The factors that may predispose to seizures are described below.

Family history
There is an increased liability to seizures in relatives of patients with epilepsy (up to 40% in the case of absence seizures). No single genetic trait can account for the vast heterogeneity of all epilepsies. The mechanism probably involves factors that alter membrane structure or function, leading to a lowered seizure threshold.

Prenatal and perinatal factors
Intrauterine infections such as rubella and toxoplasmosis can produce brain damage and neonatal seizures, as can maternal drug abuse and irradiation in early gestation. Perinatal trauma and anoxia, when sufficiently severe to cause brain injury, may also result in epilepsy.

Trauma and surgery
Severe closed or open head trauma is often followed by seizures. These can be within the first week (early) or may be delayed up to several months or years (late), when the likelihood of chronic epilepsy is greater. Surgery to the cerebral hemispheres is followed by seizures in about 10% of patients.

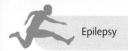

International Classification of Epileptic Seizures
Partial seizures (seizures beginning focally)
simple (consciousness not impaired) with motor symptoms with somatosensory or special sensory symptoms with autonomic symptoms with psychic symptoms
complex (with impairment of consciousness) beginning as a simple partial seizure and progressing to a   complex partial seizure impairment of consciousness at onset
partial seizure becoming secondarily generalized
Generalized seizure
absence seizure typical (petit mal) atypical
myoclonic seizure clonic seizure tonic seizure tonic-clonic seizure (grand mal) atonic seizure

Fig. 21.1 The International Classification of Epileptic Seizures.

Metabolic causes

Many electrolyte disturbances can cause neuronal irritability and seizures. Examples include hyponatremia and hypernatremia, hypocalcemia, hypomagnesemia, and hypoglycemia. Other metabolic causes include uremia, hepatic failure, acute hypoxia, and porphyria. Chronic metabolic encephalopathies produce gray-matter injury.

Toxic causes

Drugs such as phenothiazines, monoamine oxidase inhibitors, tricyclics, amphetamines, lidocaine, and nalidixic acid may provoke seizures, either in overdose or at therapeutic levels in patients with a lowered seizure threshold.

Withdrawal of antiepileptic medication and benzodiazepines may also cause seizures.

Chronic alcohol abuse is a common cause of seizures. These may occur while drinking, during abstention, or secondary to hypoglycemia.

Other toxic agents capable of causing seizures include carbon monoxide, lead, and mercury.

Infectious and inflammatory causes

Seizures may be the presenting feature or part of the course of encephalitis, meningitis, cerebral abscess, Lyme disease, or neurosyphilis and usually indicate a poorer prognosis in these conditions. High fevers secondary to non-cerebral infections in children under 5 years of age are a common cause of generalized seizures ("febrile convulsion"). These are usually self-limiting, and seizures do not tend to recur in adult life.

Vascular causes

Up to 15% of patients with cerebrovascular disease experience seizures, especially with large areas of infarction or hemorrhage. Less common vascular causes of seizures include cortical venous thrombosis and arteritis (e.g., polyarteritis nodosa).

Intracranial tumors

Sudden onset of seizures in adult life, especially if partial, should always raise the possibility of an intracranial tumor.

Hypoxia

Seizures can develop during or following respiratory or cardiac arrest, as a result of anoxic encephalopathy.

Degenerative diseases

All patients with degenerative corticoneuronal diseases of the brain have an increased risk for seizures.

Photosensitivity

Some seizure types are precipitated by flashing lights or flickering television or computer screens.

Pathophysiology

Electrical discharges between neurons are usually restricted, and produce the normal rhythms recorded on the electroencephalogram (EEG).

When a seizure occurs, large groups of neurons are activated repetitively and "hypersynchronously," with dysfunction of the inhibitory synaptic contact between neurons.

The onset of the epileptic discharge may include the whole cortex ("primary generalized"), may be confined to one area of the cortex ("partial"), or may start focally and then spread to involve the whole cortex ("secondary generalization of a partial seizure").

Clinical features

The diagnosis of epilepsy is primarily a clinical one; therefore, a detailed description of events is essential and usually requires eye-witness reports.

If an aura preceded the attack, the patient may be able to describe this, which may help localize the focus; however, it may have been forgotten as a result of retrograde amnesia.

Simple partial seizures

Simple partial seizures involve focal symptoms, most commonly motor or sensory, arising in the frontal motor or parietal sensory cortex and affecting the contralateral face, trunk, or limbs. There is no loss of awareness unless there is a subsequent spread of activity ("secondary generalization"). A structural brain lesion must be excluded.

Complex partial seizures

Complex partial seizures usually originate in the temporal lobe and involve complex auras and partial clouding of awareness. The actual attack varies between individuals (and even in the same individual) and may include *déjà vu*, depersonalization, epigastric fullness, strange tastes or smells, lip smacking, or altered emotion.

Absence seizures (petit mal)

Absence seizures have an onset between 4 and 12 years of age. The attacks may occur several times a day, with a duration of 5–15 seconds. The patient stares vacantly. There may be eye blinking. They are often diagnosed following complaints about an inattentive child with a deteriorating performance at school.

Tonic-clonic seizures (grand mal)

Tonic-clonic seizures start with a loss of consciousness, followed by the "tonic" phase, which lasts for about 10 seconds. The body is stiff; the elbows are flexed and the legs extended; breathing stops. Bladder and bowel function may be lost at the end of this phase.

Then comes the "clonic phase," which lasts for about 1–2 minutes. There is violent generalized shaking; the eyes roll; the tongue may be bitten; there is tachycardia. Breathing recommences at the end of this phase.

Following a tonic-clonic seizure, the patient is often unarousable for a variable period and awakes with confusion and headache.

History and investigations to aid diagnosis

The diagnosis of a seizure is based on the clinical history. Additional information may be provided by brain imaging, the EEG, or blood tests.

In generalized seizures, the PO_2 and pH are lowered, the creatine phosphokinase (CPK, creatine kinase, or CK) is elevated, and there is an elevation of serum prolactin.

The EEG is extremely useful if recorded during an attack, but interictal EEGs are often normal. In some cases, abnormal activity can be evoked by hyperventilation or photic stimulation (flashing light), as is often the case for absence seizures, in which there is the characteristic three-per-second spike-and-wave pattern in all leads (Fig. 19.7).

Computed tomography (CT) or magnetic resonance imaging (MRI) may reveal structural lesions that have caused the seizures, or, in temporal lobe epilepsy, may show hippocampal sclerosis.

Differential diagnosis

It is most important to distinguish epilepsy from other causes of transient focal dysfunction or loss of consciousness because of the social and economic implications when a diagnosis of epilepsy is made (e.g., inability to drive or operate certain machinery).

The most common differentials include:

- Syncope (arrhythmias, carotid sinus hypersensitivity, vasovagal attacks, postural hypotension): there is usually prodromal pallor, nausea, and sweating. Palpitations may be experienced with arrhythmias.
- Nonepileptic seizures ("psychogenic seizures"): hysterical, stress-related seizures are surprisingly common, especially in patients with known epilepsy. The following features help to

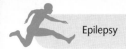

differentiate a pseudoseizure from an epileptic seizure: pupils, blood pressure, heart rate, PO_2, and pH remain unchanged; plantar responses are flexor; serum prolactin levels are normal; the EEG shows no seizure activity during the episode and no postictal slowing.

- Transient ischemic attacks can include transient loss of consciousness when the posterior circulation is involved.
- Hypoglycemia can cause behavioral disturbance and seizures.

Drug treatment

When two or more unprovoked seizures have occurred, antiepileptic treatment should be considered. Whenever possible, treatment should involve only one drug to avoid interactions and minimize side effects. Treatment is aimed at making the patient seizure-free, but this goal is not always possible.

The most common antiepileptic drugs in current clinical use include phenytoin, carbamazepine, sodium valproate, and lamotrigine. Other drugs include gabapentin, topiramate, levitiracetam, oxcarbazepine, gabitril, primidone, zonisamide, phenobarbital, and pregabalin. In general, the first-line drug for generalized epilepsy in adults is sodium valproate or lamotrigine; for absence epilepsy in children, ethosuximide; and for partial epilepsy, carbamazepine.

The drugs should be built up slowly. Measurement of blood drug concentrations is important for phenytoin, because it displays zero-order kinetics at higher doses and small increases in dose can cause it to reach toxic levels. For other drugs, therapeutic drug monitoring can be used to check compliance or to confirm clinically diagnosed toxicity.

Pharmacokinetics of antiepileptic drugs

Many of the antiepileptic drugs possess unusual pharmacokinetics (e.g., phenytoin, carbamazepine, and valproate). Care must be taken when prescribing these drugs, especially in combination, to avoid toxic levels and other adverse reactions.

Adverse effects of antiepileptic drugs

All antiepileptic drugs may produce acute dose-related, acute idiosyncratic, or chronic toxicity, and variable degrees of teratogenicity (damage to the developing fetus).

Acute toxicity

Some antiepileptic drugs cause a nonspecific encephalopathy when blood levels are high, with sedation, nystagmus, ataxia, dysarthria, and confusion. If any of these features are present, blood levels must be measured. (Note: including the active epoxide metabolite of carbamazepine.) Toxicity may also occur due to drug interactions (e.g., valproate prolongs the half-life of lamotrigine).

Idiosyncratic toxicity

Allergic skin reactions occur in up to 10% of patients on phenytoin and lamotrigine and in up to 5% on carbamazepine. Bone marrow suppression is a rare complication of carbamazepine.

Chronic toxicity

Chronic toxicity is especially associated with phenytoin and includes the development of coarsened facies, acne and hirsutism, gum hypertrophy, and peripheral neuropathy. Most antiepileptic drugs appear to have some effect on cognitive function.

Teratogenicity

Phenytoin increases the risk of major fetal malformation—including cleft lip, cleft palate, and cardiovascular anomalies—by two times. The use of sodium valproate and carbamazepine in pregnancy is associated with neural tube defects. The antiepileptic drugs also have cognitive effects on a developing fetus. Folate supplements, and early screening using ultrasound and amniocentesis (to test for alpha-fetoprotein), are indicated in such cases.

Patients with epilepsy and on treatment who wish to become pregnant should seek specialist advice before conception and require regular follow up by a neurologist during the pregnancy.

Withdrawal of antiepileptic drugs

In view of the many adverse reactions associated with antiepileptic drugs, a patient who has achieved remission for over 2 years should be considered for drug withdrawal. However, there is the risk of recurrence of seizures, especially in some forms of epilepsy, and this has important consequences for driving, employment, and self-esteem. Thus, the final decision to attempt withdrawal must be made by the patient, and if undertaken, must be carried out very slowly, with gradually decreasing doses.

Status epilepticus

Patients with status epilepticus require immediate resuscitation: establish an airway; administer oxygen (hypoxia is common); assess the circulation; set up an infusion of normal saline.

Blood tests include blood gases, glucose, electrolytes, renal and liver function, toxicology screen, and antiepileptic drug levels.

 If hypoglycemia is suspected in patients with a possible history of alcohol abuse or malnutrition, thiamine must be given with intravenous glucose, because glucose alone can precipitate Wernicke's encephalopathy.

Drug treatment

It is helpful to plan therapy in a series of progressive phases:

- Premonitory stage (0–10 minutes): rapid treatment may prevent the evolution to status. Lorazepam or diazepam can be used at this stage.
- Early status (0–30 minutes): a dose of fast-acting intravenous benzodiazepines (either lorazepam or diazepam) should be given, repeated once if seizures are not terminated. (Note: repeated doses of benzodiazepines lead to accumulation and risk of respiratory depression.)
- Established status (30–60 minutes): usually phenobarbital or phenytoin is given at this stage, as large, intravenous loading doses.

Refractory status (after 60 minutes): by this stage, anesthesia is required, with ventilation and intensive care treatment. The most commonly used agents are intravenous phenobarbital, thiopental, or propofol. EEG monitoring is very helpful. In all cases, neuromuscular blockade should be avoided if possible.

Neurosurgical treatment of epilepsy

Patients with intractable epilepsy (failure of three or more antiepileptic agents) are candidates for epilepsy surgery. Surgical treatment requires the accurate identification of a localized site of onset of seizures or the ability to disconnect epileptogenic zones and prevent spread as a palliative procedure.

The majority of the procedures undertaken in centers worldwide involve some form of temporal lobe surgery. In addition, extratemporal cortical excisions, hemispherectomies, and corpus callosotomies are carried out.

For temporal lobe surgery, the two conditions with the best surgical outcome are medial temporal sclerosis (Ammon's horn sclerosis) and an indolent glioma of the medial temporal region. Epilepsy surgery is underutilized.

The social consequences of epilepsy

Considerable social stigma is attached to a diagnosis of epilepsy.

There are implications for employment, not only in the ability to carry out certain jobs (e.g., driving or using machinery), but also because many employers are unwilling to take on persons with epilepsy.

The aim is to allow patients to lead as unrestricted a life as possible but bearing in mind some precautions, such as to avoid swimming alone or engaging in dangerous sports such as rock climbing. They should also be advised about simple domestic precautions such as not locking the bathroom door.

Driving and epilepsy

Patients who have suffered one or more seizures are restricted from holding a driver's license.

Every state regulates driver's license eligibility differently. Most require a period of remaining seizure-free before driving and completion of driving forms by physicians. In six states a physician must report patients with seizures to the motor vehicles department: California, Delaware, New Jersey, Pennsylvania, Nevada, and Oregon.

22. Headache and Craniofacial Pain

Headache is one of the most common symptoms in medicine and may account for up to 40% of neurologic consultations.

There is a great deal of overlap in the presentations of headache, and although the characteristic features of particular types of headache will be presented in this chapter, it is important to bear in mind that, in practice, symptoms are often not as clear-cut.

Tension headache

Tension headache is the most common form of headache and is experienced by most people at some point in their lives.

There is a diffuse, "band-like," dull headache, which may be accompanied by scalp tenderness and be aggravated by noise and light. It may last from hours to days. It may be infrequent or daily and is usually worse toward the end of the day. There are no abnormal physical signs.

Treatment is with reassurance, analgesia, physical treatments (massage, relaxation therapy), and antidepressants when indicated. Paradoxically, these headaches can be exacerbated by analgesic overuse (rebound headaches), especially codeine-containing drugs, and thus stopping these drugs may help.

Migraine

Migraine is a common, often familial, condition characterized by an episodic, unilateral, throbbing headache lasting 1–24 hours. It is much more common in women, especially when young. There is often a visual prodrome with fortification spectra or flashing lights.

The headache is thought to have a vascular component and to be related to the release of vasoactive substances. The level of serum 5-hydroxytryptamine (5-HT) rises with the prodromal symptoms and falls during the headache.

There are various subdivisions of migraine, although migraine with aura and migraine without aura are the most frequently encountered forms.

Migraine with aura

An aura, which is usually visual, precedes the headache. Typically, the headache is unilateral and throbbing, accompanied by nausea and vomiting, aggravated by light (photophobia) and relieved by sleep in a darkened room.

Migraine without aura

There is no aura. The headache is similar to migraine with aura but may be more indistinct and merge more with tension headache.

Basilar migraine

In basilar migraine, the prodromal symptoms result from dysfunction in the territory of the posterior cerebral circulation, with bilateral visual symptoms, ataxia, dysarthria, vertigo, limb paresthesias, and even weakness. There may be loss of consciousness prior to the onset of headache.

Hemiplegic migraine

Hemiplegic migraine is rare and involves hemiplegia that can persist for days after the headache has settled. In some cases there is an autosomal dominant transmission.

Ophthalmoplegic migraine

Extraocular palsies, usually the third nerve, occurring with a migraine constitute ophthalmoplegic migraine. This is rare and difficult to differentiate from other causes of a third nerve palsy.

Diagnosis and differential diagnosis

The diagnosis is usually made from the history, because there are usually no clinical findings in the more common forms of migraine.

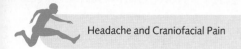

Primary headache needs to be differentiated from secondary headache due to meningitis or subarachnoid hemorrhage, both of which require prompt treatment.

Hemiplegic migraine must be differentiated from stroke or transient ischemic attacks.

Management

The patient needs to be reassured. Avoidance of any precipitating dietary factors (e.g., chocolate, cheese) may be helpful. For patients taking oral contraceptives, changing the brand or stopping the drug may be required.

During an attack
Antiemetics are often required to allow ingestion of other drugs such as simple analgesics (e.g., phenergan) or stronger analgesics (e.g., codeine-containing drugs).

Attacks may be terminated by the use of 5-HT agonists (sumatriptan, naratriptan, zolmitriptan, rizatriptan). Ergotamine is now rarely used because of more frequent side effects.

Prophylaxis
For frequent and severe attacks, regular daily treatment may be required to prevent onset. Commonly used drugs include:
- Propranolol (beta-adrenergic-receptor blocker).
- Calcium channel blockers.
- Antidepressants, especially selective serotonin-reuptake inhibitors (e.g., paxil).
- Methysergide (5-HT antagonist)—rarely used now as it causes retroperitoneal fibrosis.

Cluster headache

Cluster headache is a characteristic headache syndrome that occurs more commonly in men, with an onset in early middle life.

Features
Features of cluster headache include severe unilateral pain localized around the eye with unilateral:
- Conjunctival injection.
- Lacrimation.
- Rhinorrhea.
- With or without transient Horner's syndrome.

The headache and associated features last between 10 minutes and 2 hours, typically occurring one to three times daily in clusters lasting weeks or a few months at a time. Intervals between clusters may extend to several years. Onset of an attack is often in the early hours of the morning, waking the patient from sleep.

Treatment
Treatments used in migraine, particularly sumatriptan and ergotamine, can be helpful in cluster headache.

Specific treatments include a course of corticosteroids (e.g., 60 mg of prednisolone for 5–10 days), inhaled 100% oxygen, indomethacin and verapamil. Methysergide can be used for resistant cases, but under hospital supervision since it can cause retroperitoneal fibrosis. Lithium can be used during an acute cluster but is particularly useful if the symptoms are more chronic; however, levels need to be monitored.

Giant-cell arteritis (temporal arteritis)

Giant-cell arteritis is a granulomatous arteritis, usually affecting the superficial temporal artery in those over 60 years old.

The majority of patients experience pain over the thickened, tender, often nonpulsatile, temporal artery.

The headache is accompanied by:
- A raised erythrocyte sedimentation rate (ESR)—often marked (60–100).
- Visual loss (25% of untreated cases): amaurosis fugax (a transient ischemic attack involving the retinal vessels); permanent visual loss due to inflammation or occlusion of the ciliary or retinal vessels.
- Jaw claudication.
- Systemic features: proximal muscle pain—polymyalgia rheumatica (up to 50% of cases); weight loss; lethargy.
- Rarer complications: brainstem ischemia; cortical blindness; cranial nerve lesions; aortitis; involvement of coronary and mesenteric arteries.

Diagnosis
The diagnosis is made from the history and a raised ESR (it is rarely normal). It is confirmed by a biopsy

of the temporal artery (at least 1 cm, since the disease process may be patchy).

Treatment

Treatment is with high-dose corticosteroids (e.g., prednisolone, 60mg/day). There is a risk of blindness if treatment is delayed; hence the steroids should be started immediately, prior to the biopsy.

The dose is reduced as the ESR falls. It is usually possible to withdraw steroids slowly after several months to years.

Raised intracranial pressure

The headache of raised intracranial pressure, caused by an intracranial tumor, abscess, or other space-occupying lesion, has certain characteristic features:

- There is a generalized ache, often centered at the vertex.
- It is aggravated by bending, coughing, or straining.
- It is worse in the morning.
- It may awaken the patient from sleep.
- The severity gradually progresses.

It is accompanied by:

- Vomiting.
- Visual obscurations (transient loss of vision with sudden changes in posture).
- With or without focal neurologic signs.
- Risk of herniation—cerebellar tonsils or uncus of temporal lobe.

Imaging of the brain with computed tomography or magnetic resonance imaging is essential. Contrast may be required to visualize the lesion. (See Chapter 32 for further management of intracranial masses.)

Other neurologic causes of headache and craniofacial pain

These include:

- Intracranial hemorrhage—see Chapter 31.
- Meningitis—see Chapter 33.
- Trigeminal and postherpetic neuralgia—see Chapter 24.
- Pseudotumor cerebri.

Nonneurologic causes of headache and craniofacial pain

Local causes

Local causes include:

- Sinus disease.
- Ocular—glaucoma, refraction errors.
- Temporomandibular joint dysfunction.
- Dental disease.

Systemic causes

Headache may accompany any febrile illness, or may be a presenting feature of metabolic disease (e.g., hypoglycemia) or malignant hypertension. Certain drugs may also cause headache (e.g., nitrates, lamotrigine, caffeine).

23. Parkinson's Disease, Other Extrapyramidal Disorders, and Myoclonus

Extrapyramidal conditions cause disorders of movement, which can be broadly divided into two categories:

- Those associated with diminished movement and an increase in tone—akinetic-rigid syndromes.
- Those associated with added movements outside voluntary control—dyskinesias.

These conditions involve lesions of the basal ganglia and their connections.

Akinetic-rigid syndromes

Parkinson's disease

Parkinson's disease was first described in 1817 by James Parkinson, who named it the "shaking palsy." It is the most common of all the movement disorders. The disease is seen worldwide, with increasing incidence with age. The prevalence is 1 in 200 in those over 70 years. It is more common in men than in women.

Pathology

There is progressive degeneration of cells within the pars compacta of the substantia nigra in the midbrain (Fig. 23.1), with the appearance of eosinophilic inclusions (Lewy bodies). Minor changes may also be seen in other brainstem nuclei (striatum and globus pallidus). As a result, there is a reduction in dopamine in the striatum, disrupting the normal dopamine : acetylcholine ratio.

Etiology

The cause of Parkinson's disease is unknown. Discordance in identical twins suggests that genetic factors are not paramount. However, a consistent environmental factor has not been elucidated. Increased interest in exogenous toxins as a cause arose with the finding that drug addicts taking heroin contaminated with 1-methyl-4 phenyl-1,2,3,6-tetrahydropyridine (MPTP) developed a similar condition, with selective destruction of the nigral cells and their striatal connections.

A distinction must be made between "idiopathic Parkinson's disease" and "parkinsonism." Parkinsonism denotes a syndrome that appears clinically similar to idiopathic Parkinson's disease but has a different pathologic or etiologic basis. Causes of parkinsonism include:

- Drugs—especially dopamine antagonists (e.g., phenothiazines, reserpine, haloperidol) and the antiepileptic drug sodium valproate.
- Trauma—especially repetitive head injury (e.g., boxing).
- Cerebrovascular disease—especially lacunar infarcts of the basal ganglia.
- Toxins such as MPTP.

Clinical features

Clinical features of Parkinson's disease include the classic triad of tremor, rigidity, and bradykinesia, in association with important changes in posture and gait and a mask-like, expressionless face.

There is usually striking asymmetry in tremor and rigidity; therefore, symmetrical onset should call into question a diagnosis of idiopathic Parkinson's disease.

Tremor

This is a characteristic coarse resting tremor (4–7 Hz), which is usually decreased by action, increased with emotion, and disappears during sleep. The tremor is often "pill-rolling," with the thumb moving rhythmically backward and forward on the palmar surface of the fingers (Fig. 23.2).

Rigidity

Stiffness of the limbs can be felt throughout the range of movement and equally in the flexors and extensors. This is termed "lead-pipe" rigidity. When combined with the tremor, there is a jerky element, which is termed "cog-wheel" rigidity. The increase in tone can be felt most easily when the joint is moved slowly and steadily and can be made more apparent

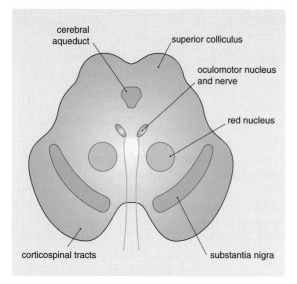

Fig. 23.1 Cross-section of the midbrain.

Differences between spasticity and rigidity	
Spasticity	**Rigidity**
lesion in upper motor neuron	lesion in basal ganglia and connections
increased tone more marked in flexors in arms and extensors in legs	increased tone equal in flexors and extensors
increased tone most apparent early during movement "clasp-knife reflex"	increased tone apparent throughout range of movement
reflexes brisk with extensor plantars	normal reflexes with flexor plantars

Fig. 23.3 The differences between spasticity and rigidity.

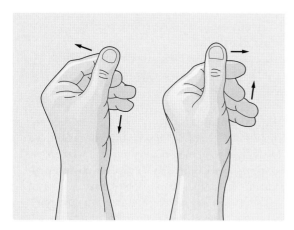

Fig. 23.2 "Pill-rolling" tremor.

when the patient is asked to voluntarily move the opposite limb (synkinesis).

The rigidity is often asymmetrical and may be very marked in the trunk (axial rigidity).

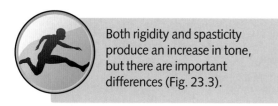

Both rigidity and spasticity produce an increase in tone, but there are important differences (Fig. 23.3).

Bradykinesia (akinesia)

Slowing and paucity of movement also occurs. In addition to the limbs, this affects the muscles of

facial expression (mask-like facies), the muscles of mastication, speech, and voluntary swallowing, and the axial muscles. There is difficulty in initiating movements and alternating movements. Turning over in bed is especially difficult.

Postural changes

The posture is characteristically stooped (Fig. 23.4), with a shuffling, festinating gait with poor arm swing. Falls are common, as the normal righting reflexes are affected. The patient falls stiffly, "like a totem pole."

Other features

Speech is altered, producing a monotonous, hypophonic dysarthria, due to a combination of bradykinesia, rigidity, and tremor. Power is normal, however in advanced disease, the slowness (akinesia) and rigidity makes testing power difficult. Sensory examination is also normal, although patients describe discomfort in the legs. Handwriting reduces in size and becomes spidery (micrographia). Constipation is usual and urinary difficulties are common, especially in men. Depression is common.

Cognitive function is preserved in the early stages, although dementia may occur late (to be differentiated from Lewy body dementia, in which Lewy bodies are found profusely in the cerebral cortex).

Natural history

Parkinson's disease progresses over a period of years. The rate of progression is highly variable, with the

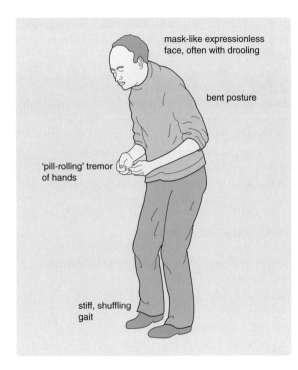

mask-like expressionless
face, often with drooling

bent posture

'pill-rolling' tremor
of hands

stiff, shuffling
gait

Fig. 23.4 Parkinsonian posture.

mildest forms running over several decades. Usually
the course is over 10–15 years, with death from
bronchopneumonia.

Differential diagnosis

The diagnosis of Parkinson's disease is a clinical one.
It must be differentiated from the other akinetic-
rigid syndromes (see later), secondary causes of
parkinsonism (drugs, cerebrovascular disease,
trauma), hypothyroidism, depression (especially in
the elderly), and diffuse multifocal brain diseases
that may have some of the features of parkinsonism.

Treatment

Drug treatment is aimed at restoring the
dopamine: acetylcholine balance caused by the
dopamine deficiency and therefore either involves
restoring dopamine or reducing acetylcholine.

Levodopa (L-dopa)

Levodopa forms the mainstay for the treatment of
most patients with Parkinson's disease. It is given in
a combined form with a peripheral decarboxylase
inhibitor (carbidopa—as Sinemet) to prevent
peripheral breakdown of the drug and to reduce the

peripheral side effects (nausea, vomiting,
hypotension).

Treatment is commenced gradually and increased
slowly until either an adequate effect is achieved or
side effects limit further increases. Levodopa
improves bradykinesia and rigidity but has a lesser
effect on tremor.

The majority of patients with Parkinson's disease
(but not other parkinsonian syndromes) initially
improve with L-dopa. However, with time the effect
becomes diminished, the duration of action of the
drug contracts, there are marked fluctuations in
symptoms, and patients experience the "on–off
syndrome." In the latter, there are marked swings
between dopa-induced dyskinesias (chorea,
dystonia) and severe and often sudden periods of
immobility ("freezing"), which may bear no
relationship to the timing of the L-dopa dose.
Consequently, L-dopa therapy should not be started
until necessary.

Dopamine agonists

Dopamine agonists are analogs of dopamine and
directly stimulate the dopamine receptors. The most
effective antiparkinsonian dopamine agonists
stimulate D_2 receptors predominantly.

Dopamine agonists have varying selectivity and
include bromocriptine, pergolide, pramipexole, and
ropinirole. Each drug has different side effects,
including nausea, dry mouth, orthostatic
hypotension, hallucinations, and psychosis.

These can be used alone, especially in younger
patients (aged less than 60 years) or to delay L-dopa
use, or as an adjunct to L-dopa.

Anticholinergic drugs

Anticholinergic drugs include bentropine and
trihexyphenidyl, which are antimuscarinic agents
that penetrate the central nervous system. They are
most effective in reducing tremor, though not so
effective for rigidity and bradykinesia. Side effects
(dry mouth, constipation, urinary retention, visual
blurring, hallucinations, and confusion) often prevent
their use, especially in the elderly.

Selegiline

Selegiline is an inhibitor of monoamine oxidase B,
thus blocking the metabolism of central dopamine.
Early use can delay the need for L-dopa, but there
may be an increased risk of cardiovascular morbidity
in advanced cases.

COMT (catechol-O-methyltransferase) antagonists

COMT antagonists are a new group of drugs. Dopamine is broken down peripherally by both decarboxylase and COMT. The rationale of these drugs is therefore to prevent the additional COMT-mediated breakdown and thus allow greater dopamine availability centrally. They are used in conjunction with L-dopa in order to reduce the L-dopa dose. Entacapone is currently the only drug in use in this group, as tolcapone has been withdrawn due to reports of death due to hepatic failure.

Surgery

Surgery is not extensively carried out but does have a place in severe cases and young patients. The techniques used include stereotactic thalamotomy for severe tremor, pallidotomy, transplantation of fetal substantia nigra, and subthalamic neurostimulators.

"Parkinson's plus" syndromes

"Parkinson's plus" syndromes have some or all of the features of idiopathic Parkinson's disease plus other features.

Progressive supranuclear palsy (Steele–Richardson–Olszewski syndrome)

Progressive supranuclear palsy may mimic Parkinson's disease in the early stages. There is marked axial rigidity, dementia, and a striking gaze palsy that initially affects vertical gaze but subsequently all the eye movements. Pseudobulbar palsy develops insidiously with dysarthria and swallowing impairment. There is usually little response to L-dopa. There is relentless progression, with a median survival of less than 6 years.

Multisystem atrophy

There are three main variants of multisystem atrophy:
- Striatonigral degeneration: picture similar to Parkinson's disease but without the tremor. There is usually no response to medication.
- Shy–Drager syndrome: parkinsonism combined with severe autonomic failure. The parkinsonian features may respond well to L-dopa, but the resulting postural hypotension often forces withdrawal of the drug.
- Olivopontocerebellar atrophy (OPCA): presentation with this condition is variable—in some patients parkinsonian features predominate, whereas in others cerebellar features are more prominent.

Other parkinsonian syndromes
Drug-induced parkinsonism

All drugs that have dopamine antagonist effects can cause a parkinsonian syndrome, usually with bradykinesia and rigidity but little tremor. The neuroleptics (phenothiazines) are a common cause. Other drugs include reserpine, butyrophenones, metoclopramide, and prochlorperazine.

Cerebrovascular disease

The pathologic basis of cerebrovascular disease causing parkinsonism is usually multifocal small-vessel disease, particularly subcortical lacunar infarcts.

Wilson's disease

Wilson's disease is an inherited autosomal recessive disorder of copper metabolism which causes copper deposition in the brain (particularly the basal ganglia), in the cornea (Kayser–Fleischer rings), and in the liver (causing cirrhosis). This is a treatable disease and the neurologic damage is reversible if caught early.

Dyskinetic syndromes

Dyskinesias can be further subdivided into:
- Tremor—rhythmic oscillation of a body part, produced by either alternating or synchronous contractions of reciprocally innervated antagonistic muscles.
- Dystonia—a disorder dominated by sustained muscle contractions, which frequently cause twisting and repetitive movements or abnormal postures. Dystonic movements may be slow and writhing. When these are distal, they are termed athetosis.
- Chorea—from the Greek word for "dance," this consists of irregular, unpredictable, brief, jerky movements that flit from one part of the body to another in a random sequence. When the movements are slower and more flowing, the term choreoathetosis is applied.
- Tics—abrupt, transient, stereotypical, coordinated movements, which vary in intensity and are repeated at irregular intervals.

- Ballism—the least common of the dyskinesias, derived from the Greek word "to throw," this involves wide-amplitude, violent, flailing movements. There is prominent involvement of proximal muscles.

Many conditions incorporate one or more of the above dyskinesias. In the following section, only the most common or important ones will be discussed.

Tremor
Benign essential tremor
Benign essential tremor is a common condition, often inherited as an autosomal dominant trait. It causes tremor at 5–8 Hz, which is usually worse in the upper limbs. The head may be tremulous (titubation) as well as the trunk. It is most apparent on posture (e.g., holding a glass) or with emotion, but is not usually present at rest, nor does it worsen on movement. Treatment is not usually necessary, but small doses of primidone or a beta blocker (e.g., propranolol) often dramatically reduce tremor.

Dystonia
Dystonia can be generalized, focal, or secondary (e.g., to drugs).

Dystonia musculorum deformans
Dystonia musculorum deformans may be inherited as an autosomal dominant or recessive gene. The latter is especially common in Ashkenazi Jews. It commences in childhood with dystonic spasms of the limbs affecting gait and posture. It gradually progresses to involve all parts of the body over one or two decades. Plateauing of symptoms or spontaneous remissions can occur. Medical treatment is often ineffective.

Dopa-responsive dystonia
Dopa-responsive dystonia is progressive dystonia affecting the lower limbs initially that has an incompletely penetrant autosomal dominant mode of transmission. There is marked diurnal variation, with symptoms worsening as the day progresses and amelioration with sleep. There is a striking and permanent response to small doses of L-dopa.

Cervical dystonia ("spasmodic torticollis")
In cervical dystonia, dystonic spasms gradually develop around the neck, usually in the third to fifth decades of life, causing the head to turn (torticollis), and be drawn backwards (retrocollis) or forwards. Patients often demonstrate a "geste antagonist"—a maneuver that stops the involuntary movement (e.g., gentle pressure with the hand on the side of the jaw). Response to drug treatment is often poor; however, the use of locally injected botulinum toxin can provide good relief.

Writer's cramp
Writer's cramp is a specific inability to perform a previously highly developed skilled movement, especially writing, due to dystonic posturing. It occurs particularly in those who spend many hours writing. Other skilled functions of the hands are normal.

Blepharospasm and oromandibular dystonia
Blepharospasm and oromandibular dystonia are related conditions and consist of spasms of forced blinking and involuntary movement of the mouth and tongue (e.g., lip smacking and protrusion of the tongue), respectively. Speech and swallowing may be affected. Blepharospasm may be stopped with regular injections of botulinum toxin into the orbicularis oculi muscles.

Chorea
Huntington's disease (Huntington's chorea)
Huntington's disease is a hereditary condition caused by an expanded trinucleotide repeat on chromosome 4. It comprises relentlessly progressive chorea and dementia, which develops in middle age, and progresses to death within 12–15 years. Other movement abnormalities may coexist. There is neuronal loss in the caudate and putamen and a reduction in GABA (gamma-aminobutyric acid) and acetylcholine levels. There is no effective treatment, although phenothiazines may reduce the chorea by causing parkinsonism. A genetic test is available for prenatal diagnosis. The use of the test in relatives of sufferers requires careful counseling, as the disease develops later in life and is fatal.

Tics
Tics are very common and usually benign.

Gilles de la Tourette syndrome
Gilles de la Tourette's is a rare syndrome in which multiple tics are accompanied by sudden explosive grunting and involuntary utterance of sexually related obscenities. It develops in childhood or

adolescence and is usually lifelong. The caudate nuclei have been implicated. Treatment with neuroleptics is sometimes helpful.

Ballism
Hemiballism
Hemiballism consists of violent flailing movements of one side of the body, caused by infarction or hemorrhage in the contralateral subthalamic nucleus.

Drug-induced movement disorders

Acute dystonic reactions
Dystonia develops in 2–5% of patients on neuroleptics or antiemetics (metoclopramide and prochlorperazine). This reaction is unpredictable and can occur even after single doses of the drugs. The range of dystonias include torticollis, oculogyric crisis, and trismus. They respond rapidly to intravenous injection of an anticholinergic drug (e.g., benztropine or diphenhydramine). Some patients on neuroleptics who develop these reactions are cotreated with an oral anticholinergic.

Drug-Induced parkinsonism
See p. 140.

Akathisia
Akathisia is a restless, repetitive, and irresistible need to move, caused by neuroleptics. It ceases with drug withdrawal.

Tardive dyskinesia
Tardive dyskinesia is a movement disorder involving the face (lip smacking, grimacing, and facial contortions), which develops after chronic exposure to neuroleptics. It may be temporarily worsened when the offending drug is stopped. Less than half the cases will eventually recover. Dystonia can also occur as a 'tardive' phenomenon.

Myoclonus

Myoclonus comprises sudden, brief, shock-like involuntary movements of single muscles or groups of muscles. These movements can arise from dysfunction of the brain or spinal cord. They do not tend to originate in the extrapyramidal system and are therefore considered separately from other movement disorders.

Myoclonus occurs as part of the normal sleep startle or hypnogogic myoclonic jerk, but also occurs as part of a wide range of disorders.

Paramyoclonus multiplex
Paramyoclonus multiplex is widespread myoclonus, usually occurring in adolescents. Seizures do not occur.

Myoclonic epilepsy
Myoclonus may be a feature of many different forms of epilepsy.

Progressive myoclonic epilepsy
Myoclonus may be combined with epilepsy and progressive dementia in several inherited metabolic diseases (e.g., Lafora body disease, cherry-red spot myoclonus syndrome, lipid-storage diseases).

Postanoxic action myoclonus
Postanoxic action myoclonus occurs following severe cerebral anoxia and is sensitive to drugs that increase the 5-HT level (e.g., fluoxetine) or berzodiazepines.

Subacute sclerosing panencephalitis
Subacute sclerosing panenecephalitis (SSPE) occurs many years after contracting measles and represents an abnormal immunological response to the measles virus. There is progressive dementia, myoclonic jerking, spasticity, and rigidity. It usually leads to death within 1–2 years.

Creutzfeldt–Jakob disease (CJD)
CJD is caused by a prion, leading to a spongiform encephalopathy with progressive dementia, myoclonus, ataxia, and death within 2 years (see Chapter 33).

24. Common Cranial Neuropathies

In this chapter, only the most common cranial neuropathies will be discussed (Fig. 24.1).

Olfactory nerve (first cranial nerve)

Common causes of either hyposmia or anosmia are nasal and sinus disease. Head injury may also cause this symptom. Rarely, a tumor may compress the olfactory bulb and tract, particularly a subfrontal meningioma.

Optic nerve (second cranial nerve)

Visual field defects
Lesions at various points in the visual pathway cause characteristic patterns of visual field loss (see Fig. 5.2).

Papilledema
Papilledema is swelling of the optic disc. Initially there is redness of the disc, with blurring of the margins and loss of retinal venous pulsation. Then there is loss of the physiologic cup, and the disc becomes engorged. There may be hemorrhages around the disc.

Causes include lesions producing raised intracranial pressure (tumors, abscess, tuberculoma) and benign intracranial hypertension. Strictly speaking, optic neuritis (see below) causes a papillitis rather than papilledema.

There is an enlargement of the blind spot but usually no visual disturbance unless the disc swelling is caused by local inflammation ("papillitis"), infiltration, or acute ischemia. Late effects of severe, prolonged papilledema include constriction of the visual fields and blindness due to infarction of the nerve.

Optic neuritis
Optic neuritis is an inflammatory optic neuropathy, most often due to multiple sclerosis. There are, however, many other causes (Fig. 24.2).

With optic neuritis (in contrast to papilledema), there is early severe visual loss (often as a central scotoma). Anterior lesions may cause swelling of the disc, but often the inflammatory process is behind the eye and is named "retrobulbar neuritis." With the latter condition, there is usually no abnormality of the disc on ophthalmoscopy.

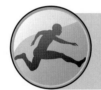

In retrobulbar neuritis, the patient sees nothing and the examiner sees nothing.

For optic neuritis caused by multiple sclerosis, the prognosis for vision is good. There is gradual improvement over a few days, weeks, or months, to relatively normal visual acuity. However, there is often a relative loss of color vision and the visual evoked potentials show delay. Other causes may result in permanent visual loss.

Optic atrophy
Optic atrophy (pale disc) may follow many different pathological processes—any of the causes in Fig. 24.2.

Oculomotor, trochlear, and abducens nerves (third, fourth, and sixth cranial nerves)

The oculomotor, trochlear, and abducens nerves are considered together, as they innervate the ocular muscles. Lesions of these nerves cause

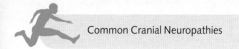

Fig. 24.1 Summary of the cranial nerves and the clinical features resulting from lesions of individual nerves.

The cranial nerves and the clinical features resulting from lesions of individual nerves		
Cranial nerve number	Cranial nerve name	Symptoms and signs caused by lesions
1	olfactory nerve	• loss of smell
2	optic nerve	• papilledema/optic neuritis • visual field defect
3	oculomotor nerve	• ophthalmoplegia with diplopia • pupillary dysfunction
4	trochlear nerve	• vertical diplopia (superior oblique palsy)
5	trigeminal nerve	• loss of sensation to the face • weakness of muscles of mastication
6	abducens nerve	• horizontal diplopia (lateral rectus palsy)
7	facial nerve	• weakness of muscles of facial expression • loss of taste (anterior two-thirds of the tongue) • hyperacusis • salivary dysfunction
8	vestibulocochlear nerve	• loss of hearing and imbalance
9	glossopharyngeal nerve	• loss of taste (posterior one-third of the tongue) • difficulties swallowing (motor and sensory loss) • salivary dysfunction • carotid sinus dysfunction
10	vagus nerve	• weakness of palate, vocal cords with swallowing difficulties
11	accessory nerve	• weakness of shrugging/ head turning
12	hypoglossal nerve	• weakness of tongue movement

ophthalmoplegia (weakness or paralysis of the relevant muscle or muscles) and diplopia (double vision).

The individual supply of these nerves is as follows:
• Trochlear nerve (fourth)—superior oblique muscle.
• Abducens nerve (sixth)—lateral rectus (lateral gaze).
• Oculomotor nerve (third)—supplies all the other muscles (medial, superior and inferior recti, inferior oblique).

Conjugate gaze

Conjugate gaze requires the coordinated functioning of both third and sixth nerves. Looking to the left requires the functioning of the left lateral rectus (sixth nerve) and the right medial rectus (third nerve). Important structures through which the information travels includes the medial longitudinal fasciculus and the parapontine reticular formation (PPRF) (Fig. 24.3).

Internuclear ophthalmoplegia

Internuclear ophthalmoplegia results from a lesion in the medial longitudinal fasciculus of the brainstem. When bilateral, it is almost pathognomonic of demyelination (multiple sclerosis). Unilateral lesions may be caused by small brainstem infarcts.

A lesion of the right medial longitudinal fasciculus causes a right internuclear ophthalmoplegia, with failure of the adduction of the right eye on attempted left lateral gaze (i.e., medial rectus

Causes of optic nerve lesions

- optic nerve compression, e.g., local or cerebral tumor, aneurysm
- papilledema—local cause
- infiltration, e.g., glioma, lymphoma
- inflammation (optic neuritis), e.g., multiple sclerosis, sarcoidosis
- ischemic, e.g., anterior ischemic optic neuropathy (AION), especially temporal arteritis
- metabolic, e.g., vitamin B_{12} deficiency
- toxins and drugs, e.g., tobacco, alcohol, methanol, ethambutol
- hereditary, e.g., Leber's optic neuropathy (mitochondrial cytopathy), part of Friedreich's ataxia
- infective, e.g., direct spread from paranasal sinuses or orbital cellulitis, syphilis
- trauma

Fig. 24.2 Causes of optic nerve lesions.

dysfunction, third nerve); in addition, there is coarse nystagmus of the left eye in abduction (Fig. 24.4).

Isolated oculomotor nerve (third nerve) lesions

The principal causes of a third nerve palsy are listed in Fig. 24.5.

Signs of a complete oculomotor nerve palsy are:
- Unilateral complete ptosis.
- Affected eye deviated in a "down-and-out" position.
- Affected pupil fixed and dilated.

Often, however, there is only partial involvement, and therefore the picture may not be as clearcut as indicated above (e.g., partial ptosis, pupil-sparing).

Pupil-sparing (i.e., the pupil is a normal size and reacts normally) indicates that the parasympathetic fibers running on the superior surface of the nerve are not involved. This is a common picture with infarction of the nerve in diabetes mellitus, but much less likely with extrinsic compressive lesions.

In a patient with a third nerve palsy, visible intorsion of the eye on attempted downward and inward gaze indicates that the fourth nerve is spared.

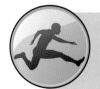

A pupil-sparing third nerve palsy is usually due to diabetes mellitus with a nerve infarct.

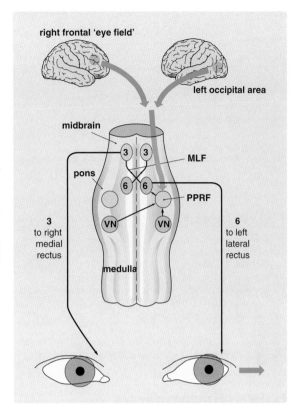

Fig. 24.3 The pathway for lateral conjugate gaze. To look left, impulses from the right frontal cortex pass to the left parapontine reticular formation (PPRF), which also has input from the vestibular nuclei and occipital cortex. Impulses generated in the left PPRF pass to both the ipsilateral (left) sixth nerve nucleus (lateral rectus, abduction) and the contralateral (right) third nerve nucleus (medial rectus, adduction). (VN, vestibular nucleus; 3, third nerve nucleus; 6, sixth nerve nucleus; MLF, medial longitudinal fasciculus.)

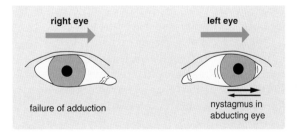

Fig. 24.4 Right internuclear ophthalmoplegia. On attempted left lateral gaze, there is failure of adduction of the right eye and coarse nystagmus of the left eye in abduction. The lesion is in the right medial longitudinal fasciculus.

Common causes of an oculomotor nerve lesion
• aneurysm of the posterior communicating artery (or internal carotid artery)—usually painful
• mononeuritis multiplex—any of the possible causes, especially diabetes (often pupil-sparing)
• midbrain infarction or tumor
• herniation of the uncus of the temporal lobe

Fig. 24.5 Common causes of an oculomotor nerve lesion.

Common causes of an abducens nerve palsy (CNVI)
• mononeuritis multiplex—any of the possible causes, especially diabetes
• multiple sclerosis
• raised intracranial pressure (false localizing sign)
• neoplasia—brainstem or local infiltration from a nasopharyngeal carcinoma
• brainstem infarction (pontine)

Fig. 24.6 Common causes of an abducens nerve palsy.

Isolated trochlear nerve (fourth nerve) palsy

Head trauma is the most common cause of an isolated fourth nerve palsy, which causes a superior oblique palsy. This results in rotation of the eye with diplopia when the patient attempts to look down and away from the affected side. The head is held tilted toward the opposite shoulder in an attempt to correct the diplopia.

Isolated abducens nerve (sixth nerve) palsy

With a sixth nerve palsy, there is failure of abduction of the affected eye due to weakness of the lateral rectus muscle. Diplopia is maximal on attempting to look laterally towards the side of the lesion.

The abducens nerve has an extremely long intracranial route from the nucleus to the lateral rectus and is often damaged by compression against the tip of the petrous bone when there is raised intracranial pressure ("false localizing sign").

The principal causes of a sixth nerve palsy are listed in Fig. 24.6.

Combined ocular palsies

Many conditions can cause combinations of third, fourth and sixth nerve palsies, with variably affected

Conditions causing combined ocular palsies	
brainstem lesions	multiple sclerosis encephalitis tumor, especially glioma, lymphoma
multiple cranial neuropathies	basal meningitis (TB, sarcoid, neoplastic, syphilis, Lyme) tumors (meningioma, lymphoma, chordoma) cavernous sinus thrombosis
neuromuscular disorders	myasthenia gravis botulinum toxin injection
ocular muscle disorders	thyroid eye disease orbital myositis infiltration, e.g., lymphoma rare ocular myopathies

Fig. 24.7 Conditions causing combined ocular palsies.

pupils and eyelids (ptosis). Some of the more common causes are listed in Fig. 24.7, including conditions that are not neuropathies but produce similar clinical pictures.

Trigeminal nerve (fifth cranial nerve)

The trigeminal nerve is mainly sensory and supplies the sensation to the face. The motor fibers supply the muscles of mastication.

The sensory fibers are divided into three branches:
• Ophthalmic (V_1)—which also supplies the cornea and takes part in the corneal reflex.
• Maxillary (V_2).
• Mandibular (V_3).

A lesion of the trigeminal nerve involving all segments will cause unilateral touch, pain, and temperature sensory loss to the face, tongue, and buccal mucosa, with reduction in the corneal reflex on the affected side. There will also be deviation of the jaw toward the side of the lesion when the mouth is opened.

The causes of a trigeminal nerve palsy are listed, according to anatomic site, in Fig. 24.8.

Trigeminal neuralgia (tic douloureux)

Trigeminal neuralgia occurs mostly in the elderly and consists of severe paroxysms of electric-shock-like

Causes of trigeminal nerve palsy according to site (CNV)	
brainstem (nuclei and connections)	multiple sclerosis infarction brainstem gliomas syringobulbia
cerebellopontine angle	acoustic neuroma meningioma
cavernous sinus	internal carotid aneurysm meningioma cavernous sinus thrombosis carotico-cavernous fistula extension of pituitary tumour
root and peripheral branches of trigeminal nerve	herpes zoster (shingles) neoplastic infiltration idiopathic trigeminal neuralgia

Fig. 24.8 Causes of trigeminal nerve palsy according to site.

Causes of facial weakness (CNVII)	
pons (there may be associated sixth nerve palsy (lateral rectus palsy), involvement of the PPRF (failure of conjugate gaze towards the lesion), and corticospinal tracts (contralateral hemiparesis)	• demyelination—multiple sclerosis • vascular lesions • pontine tumors, e.g., glioma
cerebellopontine angle (see later text)	• acoustic neuroma • meningioma • basal meningitis (TB, sarcoid, syphilis, Lyme disease, neoplastic)
within the petrous temporal bone (the geniculate ganglion lies at the genu; fibers join the facial nerve in the chorda tympani carrying taste from the anterior two-thirds of the tongue (lesion causes loss of taste); the nerve to stapedius leaves distal to the genu (lesion causes hyperacusis)	• Bell's palsy—see p. 148 • middle ear infection • trauma • herpes zoster • (Ramsay-Hunt syndrome) • tumors, e.g., glomus tumor
within the face (the branches emerge from the stylomastoid foramen and pierce the parotid gland to supply the muscles of facial expression)	• parotid gland tumors • mumps • sarcoidosis
other causes of facial weakness (often bilateral)	• mononeuritis multiplex • Guillain Barré syndrome • motor neuron disease • Myasthenia Gravis • myotonic dystrophy • facio-scapulo-humeral muscular dystrophy

Fig. 24.9 Causes of facial weakness according to site.

pain, usually in the V_3 and V_2 divisions of the trigeminal nerve. The paroxysms are usually stereotyped and can be triggered by certain stimuli (e.g., washing the face, shaving, cold wind, eating, or touching a particular position on the face).

Physical examination is normal.

The mechanism in most cases is believed to be local irritation of the nerve by the adjacent arterial vessel.

Spontaneous remissions for months or years can occur. Treatment is usually with carbamazepine or gabapentin (acting as membrane stabilizers). These do not always work and surgical intervention may be required, although the success of these procedures is limited.

Postherpetic neuralgia

Herpes zoster (shingles) may involve the trigeminal nerve, especially the ophthalmic division (V_1). There is often subsequent pain within the distribution of this division.

Facial nerve (seventh cranial nerve)

The facial nerve is mainly motor, supplying the muscles of facial expression. However, in addition, it has a sensory component, subserving taste from the anterior two-thirds of the tongue, and a parasympathetic component to the lacrimal, submaxillary, and submandibular glands (lacrimation and salivation). The most common cause of facial weakness is a supranuclear lesion (i.e., in the cerebral hemisphere), such as stroke or tumor, causing an upper motor neuron picture.

Other causes of facial weakness are listed anatomically in Fig. 24.9.

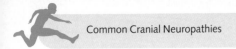

Bell's palsy

Bell's palsy consists of an acute lower motor neuron facial palsy, usually unilateral, that is of uncertain etiology but appears to cause inflammation of the facial nerve within the petrous temporal bone.

It may be preceded by a history of aching around the ear in the 24 hours before onset. The palsy is usually complete within a few hours. There should be no sensory loss in the face.

In most cases, the cause is not found. In others, causes include diabetes, mononeuritis multiplex, sarcoidosis, and Lyme disease.

The prognosis is usually extremely good, with 80% of patients making a full recovery within 2–8 weeks. If recovery is delayed, the ultimate degree of recovery is often incomplete and may be accompanied by synkinesis or "crocodile tears."

A short course of high-dose steroids within the first week is controversial, but the current thinking is that this may speed the recovery. Surgery may be required for corneal exposure and synkinesis.

> The muscles of the upper part of the face are supplied bilaterally from the motor cortex. An upper motor neuron lesion (i.e., above the level of the facial nucleus in the pons), such as a stroke or tumor, will cause unilateral weakness of the lower half of the face and spare eye closure and forehead movement. Weakness unilaterally of all the facial muscles (upper and lower face) is caused by a lower motor neuron lesion (i.e., facial nucleus or nerve) (see Fig. 17.8).

Vestibulocochlear nerve (eighth cranial nerve)

The combined vestibulocochlear nerve is responsible for hearing and balance. Lesions cause deafness, tinnitus, loss of balance, vertigo (with or without vomiting), and nystagmus.

Neurologic causes of deafness and vertigo	
brainstem	demyelination (multiple sclerosis) infarction
eighth nerve	acoustic neuroma basal meningitis trauma
end organ disease	degenerative syndromes vascular including vasculitis Ménière's disease infection (herpes zoster, mumps, etc.) benign positional vertigo

Fig. 24.10 Neurologic causes of deafness and vertigo.

Causes of deafness and vertigo are listed in Fig. 24.10.

Cerebellopontine angle lesions

The most common lesions in the cerebellopontine angle are an acoustic neuroma (a benign schwannoma of the eighth cranial nerve), and a meningioma. Other causes include metastases and other tumors. Bilateral acoustic neuromas may be found in association with neurofibromatosis type 2.

Because of the anatomy of this region (see Fig. 32.2), there is also involvement of the fifth and seventh cranial nerves and cerebellar connections. Occasionally, the sixth cranial nerve is involved.

The resulting clinical picture is of unilateral deafness, tinnitus, vertigo (with or without nystagmus), loss of facial sensation (plus corneal reflex), weakness of muscles of facial expression, and ataxia. A lateral rectus palsy may also be seen.

Diagnosis requires imaging, preferably with magnetic resonance imaging type, and treatment is surgical.

Ménière's disease

Ménière's disease comprises paroxysmal attacks of deafness, tinnitus, and severe vertigo. Ultimately, deafness becomes permanent and vertigo ceases, although the condition may remit at an earlier stage. Treatment is with vestibular sedatives. Salt restriction and diuretics may be helpful.

Benign positional vertigo

Benign positional vertigo comprises transient vertigo precipitated by head movements. Symptoms can be reproduced with nystagmus using Hallpike's maneuver (tilting down and turning the patient's head suddenly from a lying position). Treatment is with vestibular sedatives and vestibular exercises.

The lower cranial nerves— glossopharyngeal (ninth), vagus (tenth), accessory (eleventh), and hypoglossal (twelfth)

Isolated palsies of the lower cranial nerves are rare. Combined palsies, especially involving the ninth, tenth, and twelfth nerves, produce "bulbar palsies" and are found with:

- Motor neuron disease.
- Brainstem vascular disease.
- Tumors—brainstem; nasopharyngeal; skull base; glomus tumor.
- Polyneuropathy (e.g., Guillain Barré syndrome).
- Syringobulbia.
- Trauma.

25. Diseases Affecting the Spinal Cord (Myelopathy)

Anatomy of the spinal cord

The spinal cord in the adult extends from the top of the C1 vertebra to the bottom of the body of the L1 vertebra, where it is known as the conus medullaris (Fig. 25.1). It is continuous with the medulla oblongata above and the filum terminale, a fibrous band with little neural tissue, below.

The spinal cord, cauda equina, and filum terminale, down to the S2 level, is surrounded by the thick tube of dura mater, which is separated from the fine arachnoid mater by the subdural space. The arachnoid mater is separated from the pia mater, which invests the spinal cord and nerve roots, by the subarachnoid space.

When cut in cross-section, the spinal cord appears as in Fig. 25.2. It contains the central grey matter, consisting of neuronal cell bodies, and the peripheral white matter, which contains the ascending and descending fiber pathways. The ascending pathways relay sensory information from the periphery to the brain, and the descending fibers relay motor instructions *from* the brain. Different pathways have specific positions within the spinal cord and each carries specific information (see Fig. 25.2).

Most of the pathways cross over at some point in their ascent or descent. It is clinically important to know these sites, as particular syndromes result from interruption of the pathways.

Major pathways in the spinal cord

Pain and temperature

Segmental information concerning pain and temperature enters the spinal cord and crosses over to the opposite side of the cord almost immediately, to join the spinothalamic tract. This pathway runs anterolaterally in the spinal cord (see Fig. 25.2).

A lesion of the spinothalamic tract on one side will result in loss of pain and temperature contralaterally, below the level of the lesion.

Proprioception (joint-position sense) and vibration

Segmental information concerning proprioception and vibration enters the spinal cord and remains on the same side, joining the dorsal (posterior) columns. The posterior columns comprise the fasciculus cuneatus and the fasciculus gracilis and lie posteriorly in the spinal cord (see Fig. 25.2). The pathway then crosses over in the medulla. The nucleus cuneatus and the nucleus gracilis are positioned just before the crossover, and form a synapse for this pathway. The cuneatus conveys information from the upper levels of the spinal cord, and the gracilis from the lower levels.

A lesion of the dorsal columns on one side will result in loss of proprioception and vibration ipsilaterally, below the level of the lesion.

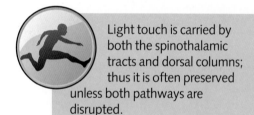

Light touch is carried by both the spinothalamic tracts and dorsal columns; thus it is often preserved unless both pathways are disrupted.

Spinocerebellar tracts

The unconscious component of proprioception is carried within the spinocerebellar tracts and enables one to walk and perform other subconscious acts. The tracts lie laterally in the spinal cord (see Fig. 25.2). Unlike other sensory pathways, which cross the midline, the spinocerebellar tracts remain ipsilateral and end in the cerebellum.

Motor pathways

The corticospinal tracts begin in the motor area of the cerebral cortex and descend ipsilaterally. They then cross in the medulla (pyramidal decussation) and descend laterally in the spinal cord (see Fig. 25.2). The tracts synapse segmentally in the anterior

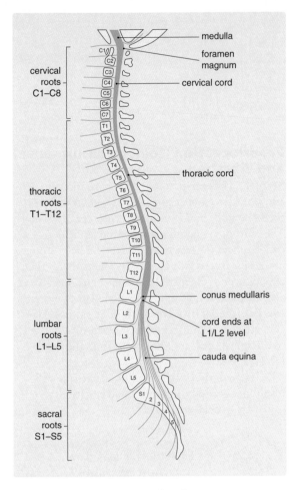

Fig. 25.1 Anatomy of the spinal cord.

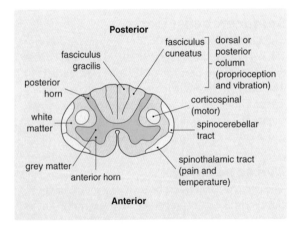

Fig. 25.2 A cross-section of the cervical spinal cord, showing the positions of the major pathways.

horn of the spinal cord (see Fig. 13.1), just prior to leaving the cord. All the connections above this level (i.e., cerebral cortex to the anterior horn) are termed the upper motor neuron, whereas the cell body (neuron) in the anterior horn (anterior horn cell) and all connections distal to this (peripheral nerve) are termed the lower motor neuron (see Fig. 13.1).

A lesion of the corticospinal tract on one side of the spinal cord will cause an ipsilateral upper motor neuron defect (spastic paresis, brisk reflexes, and an extensor plantar response).

Causes of spinal cord disease

Trauma
Transection of the cord

Spinal cord transection is usually the result of trauma, with anterior dislocation of one vertebra on another, often with fracture. It causes loss of all motor, sensory, autonomic, and sphincteric function below the level of the lesion either immediately if complete, or within hours, secondary to edema, if incomplete.

Subsequently, there are two stages:

- Spinal shock—there is loss of all reflex activity below the level of the lesion, with flaccid limbs, atonic bladder with overflow incontinence, atonic bowel, gastric dilatation, and loss of genital reflexes and vasomotor control.
- Heightened reflex activity—this occurs after about 1–2 weeks, with spasticity of the limbs with hyperactive reflexes and extensor plantar responses, spastic bladder (small capacity with urgency, frequency, and automatic emptying), and hyperactive autonomic function (sweating and vasomotor).

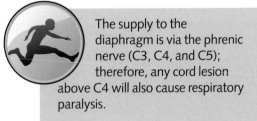

The supply to the diaphragm is via the phrenic nerve (C3, C4, and C5); therefore, any cord lesion above C4 will also cause respiratory paralysis.

Differential diagnosis

In the absence of trauma, similar symptoms and signs of a very severe cord lesion should make one consider the following:

- Ischemic infarction of the cord—occlusion of a major segmental artery; dissecting aortic aneurysm; vasculitis; atherosclerosis of the collateral arterial vessels; anterior spinal artery thrombosis.
- Hemorrhage into the spinal cord from an arteriovenous malformation; epidural or subdural hemorrhage.
- Acute necrotizing or demyelinating myelopathy—though usually subacute.
- Epidural abscess.

Treatment

The treatment of spinal fracture and dislocation is mainly orthopedic, and the reduction of edema with immediate administration of high-dose corticosteroids.

Cord compression

Depending on the site of compression, various clinical pictures may arise:

- Paraparesis.
- Tetraparesis.
- Brown–Séquard syndrome (unilateral cord compression).

They may develop rapidly or slowly, over months to years, depending on the cause.

Bilateral upper motor neuron signs in the legs (with or without arms) with no cranial nerve signs usually indicates spinal cord pathology. The lesion must be above the body of L1, as the spinal cord ends at this level and lesions below this level involve the cauda equina and so cause lower motor neuron signs.

Paraparesis (spastic paraparesis or paraplegia)

Paraparesis indicates bilateral upper motor neuron damage involving both corticospinal tracts. There is spasticity in both legs—increased tone, pyramidal distribution weakness, increased reflexes, and extensor plantar responses—and abdominal reflexes may be absent (Fig. 25.3). This pattern often produces a sensory level which approximates the level of injury. Sphincter dysfunction may be present. It is usually caused by a lesion in the thoracic cord.

Tetraparesis (spastic tetraparesis, tetraplegia, quadraparesis, quadraplegia)

Tetraparesis produces the same clinical picture as paraparesis but involves the arms, as well as the legs, bilaterally. This is usually caused by a lesion in the cervical cord or rarely the brainstem.

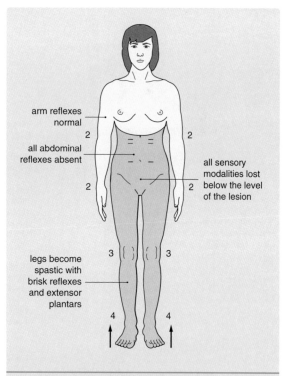

arm reflexes normal

all abdominal reflexes absent

all sensory modalities lost below the level of the lesion

legs become spastic with brisk reflexes and extensor plantars

2, normal reflex; 3, increased reflex; 4, pathologically brisk reflex with clonus; ↑, extensor plantar

Fig. 25.3 Clinical signs of cord compression caused by a lesion of the thoracic cord (at the T7 level spastic paraparesis).

Brown–Séquard syndrome (unilateral lesion of the cord)

Brown–Séquard syndrome is rare in its pure form, but partial forms are more common. The pure Brown–Séquard clinical picture (Fig. 25.4) consists of an ipsilateral spastic leg (with or without arm) with brisk reflexes and an extensor plantar response, ipsilateral loss of joint-position sense and vibration (dorsal columns), and contralateral loss of pain and temperature (spinothalamic tracts cross at their level of entry) (see Fig. 14.1).

Causes

The causes of these clinical pictures include:

- Trauma.
- Disc lesions.
- Spinal cord tumors (primary, metastatic, or myeloma).
- Inflammatory lesions (epidural abscess, tuberculoma, granuloma).
- Epidural hemorrhage.

Disc protrusion

The most common cause of disc disease results from spondylosis, which describes the degenerative changes within vertebrae and intervertebral discs that occur during aging or secondary to trauma or rheumatological disease (Fig. 25.5). Usually, discs protrude laterally and cause compression of the roots, resulting in a lower motor neuron lesion. However, discs can protrude centrally and posteriorly, resulting in cord compression, which causes a spastic paraparesis (usually thoracic disc) or tetraparesis (cervical disc), with variable sensory loss and sphincter dysfunction. There may also be signs of lateral root compression.

Spinal cord tumors

Spinal cord tumors can be:

- Intramedullary (within the spinal cord)—usually malignant (e.g., glioma, causing an intrinsic cord lesion).
- Intradural (on the surface of the cord arising from the meninges [meningioma] or spinal root [neurofibroma])—usually benign.

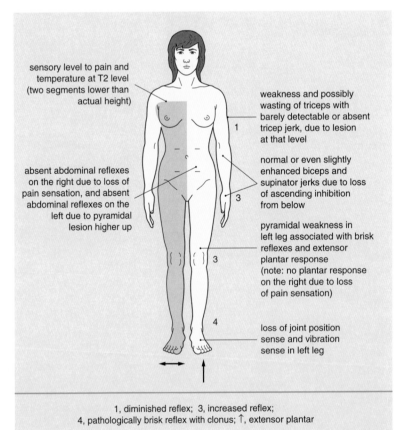

sensory level to pain and temperature at T2 level (two segments lower than actual height)

weakness and possibly wasting of triceps with barely detectable or absent tricep jerk, due to lesion at that level

absent abdominal reflexes on the right due to loss of pain sensation, and absent abdominal reflexes on the left due to pyramidal lesion higher up

normal or even slightly enhanced biceps and supinator jerks due to loss of ascending inhibition from below

pyramidal weakness in left leg associated with brisk reflexes and extensor plantar response (note: no plantar response on the right due to loss of pain sensation)

loss of joint position sense and vibration sense in left leg

1, diminished reflex; 3, increased reflex; 4, pathologically brisk reflex with clonus; ↑, extensor plantar

Fig. 25.4 Clinical signs of a Brown–Séquard lesion at level C7–C8 on the left.

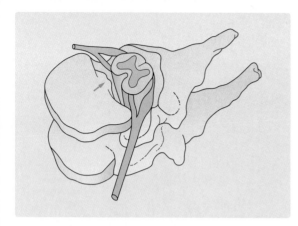

Fig. 25.5 Central disc protrusion.

- Extradural (in the epidural space)—usually manifestations of multifocal systemic neoplasia (e.g., metastatic carcinoma, lymphoma, myeloma) or can be other mass lesions (e.g., abscess, lipoma).

Inflammatory lesions
Spinal cord compression can be caused by:
- Epidural abscess (rare).
- Tuberculoma.

Epidural abscesses are most often caused by *Staphylococcus aureus*. The organism usually reaches the cord via the bloodstream but may spread directly (e.g., from osteomyelitis in a vertebra). There is fever, severe back pain with paraparesis (or tetraparesis), with or without root lesions. Diagnosis is made with magnetic resonance imaging (MRI) and lumbar puncture. Treatment is with appropriate antibiotics and surgery if necessary and treatment of the underlying source of infection.

Tuberculoma is a frequent cause of cord compression in areas where tuberculosis (TB) is common (e.g., India, Pakistan, Africa) and in areas with high immigrant populations (e.g., New York City), and often occurs in the absence of pulmonary disease. There may be destruction of vertebral bodies and spread of infection along the extradural space. This results in cord compression and paraparesis (Pott's paraplegia). Signs of a TB meningitis may coexist. Diagnosis requires a high index of suspicion. The tuberculoma can be picked up on MRI, and tubercles may be seen or grown from samples of cerebrospinal fluid. Treatment is with high-dose antituberculous therapy, which is continued for at least 9 months, and judicious use of corticosteroids for edema.

Epidural hemorrhage and hematoma
Epidural hemorrhage and hematoma are rare sequelae of anticoagulant therapy, bleeding diatheses, and trauma. A rapidly progressive cord lesion results.

Vascular cord lesions
Anterior spinal artery occlusion
This is described in Chapter 31.

Transverse myelitis
Transverse myelitis is a broad term used to describe inflammation of the cord with resultant paraparesis (or tetraparesis), arising due to a wide range of diseases:
- Multiple sclerosis.
- Viral infection.
- Connective tissue diseases (e.g., systemic lupus erythematosus).
- Syphilis.

Metabolic and toxic cord disease
Subacute combined degeneration of the cord
Subacute combined degeneration of the cord is the most important example of metabolic disease affecting the spinal cord and is caused by deficiency of vitamin B_{12}. The deficiency may result from nutritional deficiency (especially vegans), pernicious anemia, gastrectomy, or disease of the terminal ileum (e.g., Crohn's disease, "blind-loop" syndrome). Up to 25% of patients with neurologic damage caused by vitamin B_{12} deficiency do not have hematologic abnormalities (i.e., macrocytic megaloblastic anemia).

 There are only a few causes of absent ankle jerks (i.e., lower motor neuron) and extensor plantar responses (i.e., upper motor neuron). These include:
- Combined pathology (e.g., cervical spondylosis and peripheral neuropathy).
- Motor neuron disease.
- Conus lesions.
- Subacute combined degeneration of the cord (vitamin B_{12}).
- Friedreich's ataxia.
- Tabes dorsalis (neurosyphilis).

Treatment is with vitamin B_{12}, but this may not significantly improve the spinal cord damage. However, the condition can be made dramatically worse by giving folic acid.

This condition causes damage to the peripheral nerves, dorsal columns, and corticospinal tracts bilaterally. In addition there may be optic atrophy and a mild dementia. The resulting classic syndrome is of a peripheral neuropathy, a spastic paraparesis, and a sensory ataxia due to loss of joint-position sense. The full picture of an upper motor neuron lesion in the legs is prevented by the peripheral neuropathy (i.e., there is usually loss of ankle jerks), but the plantar responses are usually extensor.

Intrinsic cord lesions

The signs of an intrinsic cord lesion may be caused by a tumor or by a syrinx.

Syringomyelia and syringobulbia

Syringomyelia and syringobulbia are caused by a fluid-filled cavity (syrinx) within the spinal cord and brainstem, respectively.

The cavitation of the cervical cord is associated, in the majority of cases, with a congenital abnormality of the foramen magnum, usually a mild Arnold–Chiari malformation, with the cerebellar tonsils lying in the posterior foramen magnum. It can also arise because of an intrinsic tumor or following trauma.

Clinically, there is an evolving picture as the expanding cavity damages the various neurons and pathways (Fig. 25.6):

> In intrinsic cord lesions there is usually sacral sparing (i.e., preservation of pain and temperature sensation in the sacral dermatomes), since the ascending spinothalamic fibers from the sacrum lie peripherally and tend to be the last that are affected by the expanding cavity.

- Pain in the upper limbs is often an early feature, which may be exacerbated by coughing or straining.

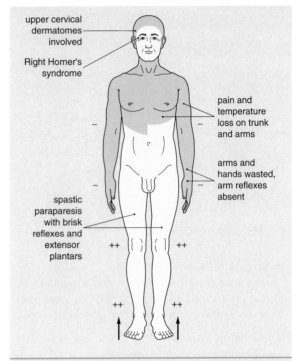

−, absent reflex; ++, normal or increased reflex; ↑, extensor plantar

Fig. 25.6 The evolving pattern of an intrinsic central cord lesion. This pattern might be seen with syringomyelia and intrinsic cord tumors (e.g., glioma, ependymoma, and astrocytoma).

- Dissociated spinothalamic sensory loss (i.e., loss of pain and temperature but preservation of touch and pressure, occurs in a "cape-like" distribution). This can extend to the head to include a "helmet" distribution.
- There is unilateral or bilateral Horner's syndrome (miosis, ptosis, and enophthalmos) due to damage to sympathetic fibers.
- There is wasting and weakness of the small muscles of the hand (anterior horn cells).
- Spastic paraparesis develops only after the cavity is markedly distended.
- Ultimately, the posterior columns may also become affected.

With syringobulbia, there is also:
- Bilateral wasting and weakness of the tongue.
- Hearing loss.
- Vestibular involvement with nystagmus.
- Facial sensory loss.

26. Motor Neuron Disease

Anatomy of the motor system

The motor cortex, situated in the precentral gyrus of the frontal cortex, contains the giant pyramidal cells of Betz. The cells of the motor cortex are arranged as a map of the body, "homunculus" (see Fig. 13.1).

The fibers pass from the motor cortex and terminate on the motor nuclei of the cranial nerves and the anterior horn cells of the spinal cord. The majority of these fibers of the "pyramidal" system cross (decussate) in the medulla to form the lateral corticospinal tracts, explaining why lesions in one cortex cause a contralateral deficit. A small proportion of the fibers remain uncrossed—the anterior corticospinal tracts.

The components rostral to the cranial nerve nuclei and anterior horn cells are within the central nervous system (CNS) and are termed the upper motor neuron (UMN), whereas those that are caudal are termed the lower motor neuron (LMN). Features of upper and lower motor neuron defects are listed in Fig. 26.1.

The individual components of the LMN include the cell body (anterior horn cell), which lies within the CNS, and its long process and the axon, the viability of which depends on the cell body. The anterior horn cell with its axon is termed the alpha motor neuron. Each alpha motor neuron extends peripherally to innervate a variable number of muscle fibers (from 20 to over 1,000). The alpha motor neuron with the muscle fibers it supplies is termed a motor unit.

In addition to the alpha motor neurons, there are smaller cell bodies that project into the anterior root and innervate the intrafusal muscle fibers of muscle spindles. These are called gamma motor neurons.

Types of motor neuron disease (MND)

MND is a disease in which there is progressive degeneration of motor neurons in the cortex and in the anterior horns of the spinal cord, and degeneration of the somatic motor nuclei of the cranial nerves within the brainstem. There is usually relentless progression of the disease to death within 1–5 years.

Depending on the distribution of involvement, the disease is subdivided into three main clinical groups and a possible, more controversial, fourth. However, these categories do not represent distinct etiologic or pathologic mechanisms, and often with time the clinical features of all the groups merge.

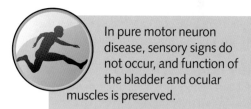

In pure motor neuron disease, sensory signs do not occur, and function of the bladder and ocular muscles is preserved.

Amyotrophic lateral sclerosis (ALS)

ALS is often used synonymously with MND. It presents with a mixture of UMN and LMN signs in the limbs—e.g., spastic tetraparesis with brisk reflexes (UMN), in association with marked wasting and fasciculations (LMN) (see Fig. 26.1). There may also be mixed bulbar features present. ("Amyotrophic" = muscle atrophy; "lateral sclerosis" = disease of lateral corticospinal tracts.)

Progressive muscular atrophy (PMA)

PMA is associated with LMN signs (wasting, weakness, and fasciculations, although tendon reflexes are usually preserved), which often begin asymmetrically in the small muscles of the hands or feet and spread. This form often progresses to involve UMN signs with time.

Progressive bulbar and pseudobulbar palsy

"Bulbar" involves the LMN; "pseudobulbar," the UMN (extra "u" in "pseudo" for underline{u}pper).

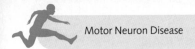

Features of upper and lower motor neuron defects	
Upper motor neuron defect	**Lower motor neuron defect**
spastic paralysis	flaccid paralysis
no significant muscle atrophy	significant muscle atrophy
no fasciculations	fasciculations present
brisk reflexes	reduced or absent reflexes
extensor plantar response (Babinski)	plantar response flexor or absent

Fig. 26.1 Features of upper and lower motor neuron defects.

The lower cranial nerve nuclei and their supranuclear connections are involved in these variants of the disease. Patients present with dysarthria, dysphagia, nasal regurgitation, choking, and dysphonia ("Donald Duck" voice). They may have wasting and fasciculation of the tongue.

Primary lateral sclerosis

Primary lateral sclerosis is somewhat more controversial as a subgroup of MND. This is a purely UMN disease, and the diagnosis can be made only after other conditions are excluded. Some patients have been known to progress to a more classic ALS-type picture.

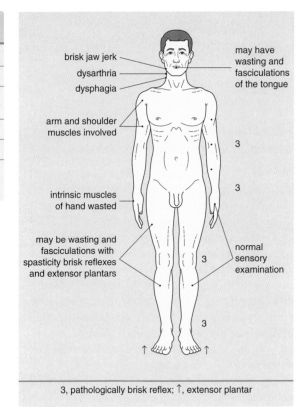

Fig. 26.2 Clinical findings in a patient with classic amyotrophic lateral sclerosis are a mixture of upper and lower motor neuron signs. There is often a mixed bulbar and pseudobulbar picture (e.g., wasted, fasciculating tongue with a spastic palate), which may remain isolated or be the presenting feature of ALS.

Epidemiology

The majority of cases of MND are sporadic; however, 5–10% are familial. The most common familial form is due to abnormal expression of the superoxide dismutase-1 gene (SOD-1) found on chromosome 21. In the remaining familial cases, the mutation is unknown.

Sporadic MND has an incidence of about 1 in 100,000. The incidence increases with age, with a peak between 60 and 70 years of age. There are endemic areas where the incidence is much higher (e.g., Guam), but it is uncertain as to whether this represents a familial form or whether it is due to some environmental factor (e.g., cycad nut).

The mean survival in patients with MND is 3 years; however, those with bulbar onset have a shorter life expectancy because aspiration pneumonia is more common.

Men are more commonly affected than women, with a ratio of 1.5:1. However, the bulbar form is slightly more common in women.

Differential diagnosis

The differential diagnosis depends on the mode of presentation:

Amyotrophic lateral sclerosis

Differential diagnoses for ALS include conditions that present with a mixture of UMN and LMN signs:
- Cervical spondylosis—combination of spinal cord compression (UMN), root compression, and anterior horn cell loss (LMN).
- Spinal tumors—reason as for cervical spondylosis.

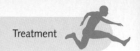

- Hyperthyroidism or hyperparathyroidism—wasted, fasciculating muscles (LMN) with brisk reflexes (UMN).
- Infections: HIV, Lyme disease, HTLV-1, syphilis.
- Toxins: mercury, lead.
- Other: muscular dystrophy, postpolio syndrome, multiple sclerosis.

Progressive muscular atrophy

Differential diagnoses for PMA include conditions with LMN signs only:

- Spinal muscular atrophy (SMA)—a heterogeneous hereditary condition with anterior horn cell loss.
- Postpolio syndrome—progressive weakness and wasting 30–40 years after having had polio, which usually affects limbs not involved in the initial disease. The exact cause is uncertain, but it does not involve reactivation of the poliomyelitis virus.
- Poliomyelitis (new onset is rare in the U.S.).
- Multifocal motor neuropathy with conduction block—autoimmune condition with high levels of anti-GM1 antibody. This is treatable with intravenous immunoglobulin and immunosuppression.
- Acute intermittent porphyria.
- Lead neuropathy.

Pseudobulbar palsy

Differential diagnoses for pseudobulbar palsy include:

- Cerebrovascular disease.
- Multiple sclerosis.
- Brainstem tumors.

Diagnosis

The diagnosis is made clinically and supported by electromyography (EMG), which shows the presence of denervation in the muscles supplied by more than one spinal region (see Chapter 19).

Other conditions must be excluded if suspected.

Treatment

There is no cure for MND. The diagnosis should be carefully and fully discussed with the patient and caregivers. Ideally, there should be counseling and multidisciplinary support. It is important to establish a living will.

Drug treatment

The newly introduced drug riluzole has been shown to increase survival by 3–6 months, but it has no effect on disability. Riluzole reduces glutamate release.

Many other drug trials are in progress and include the use of insulin-like growth factor-1 (IGF-1; Cephalon).

Symptomatic treatment

Symptomatic treatment is of paramount importance in MND and includes:

- Speech therapy and communication aids.
- Ventilatory support.
- Altered food consistency for safe swallowing, and ultimately, in some cases, a percutaneous endoscopic gastrotomy (PEG).
- Physiotherapy, splints, walking aids, and wheelchairs.
- Adaptations to allow patients to stay at home.
- Full palliative care in the terminal stages.

27. Radiculopathy and Plexopathy

Anatomy

Thirty paired spinal nerve roots provide the means of entry and exit from the central nervous system (CNS).

The dorsal root contains the sensory (afferent) fibers arising from sensory receptors in the periphery, as well as the sensory cell body, termed the dorsal root ganglion (Fig. 27.1). The ventral (anterior) root contains the motor (efferent) fibers. As mentioned in Chapter 26, the motor cell body lies within the anterior horn of the spinal cord (see Fig. 27.1). The dorsal and ventral roots lie within the spinal subarachnoid space and come together at the intervertebral foramen to become the spinal nerve.

The spinal roots and nerves are named by the vertebral level at which they emerge from the spinal cord. In the cervical region, the roots exit above each vertebral body and there are thus eight cervical roots (C1–C8) although only seven cervical vertebrae; in contrast, at all other levels, the roots emerge below the respective vertebral body, i.e. T1–T12, L1–L5 (see Fig. 25.1).

The spinal nerves, after emerging from the intervertebral foramina, pass into the brachial plexus to supply the upper limb or into the lumbosacral plexus to supply the lower limb.

The brachial plexus lies in the posterior triangle of the neck, between scalenius anterior and scalenius medius, and is derived from the C5–T1 roots. At the root of the neck, the plexus lies behind the clavicle. The plexus gives off several motor branches before forming the "cords" and ultimately becomes the median, ulnar, and radial nerves (see Fig. 13.5).

The lumbosacral plexus is subdivided into the lumbar plexus (T12–L5) and the sacral plexus (L4–S3) (see Fig. 13.6). The lumbar plexus is located in the psoas muscle and forms the femoral nerve (L2–L4); the sacral plexus is on the posterior wall of the pelvis and forms the common peroneal nerve (L4–L5, S1–S2 posterior divisions) and the tibial nerve (L4–L5, S1–S2 anterior division), which unite to form the sciatic nerve.

Radiculopathy (nerve root lesions)

Causes
Causes of radiculopathy include:
- Cervical and lumbar spondylosis (disc prolapse, degenerative changes, osteophytes).
- Trauma.
- Tumors (e.g., neurofibroma, metastases).
- Herpes zoster (shingles).
- Meningeal inflammation.
- Arachnoiditis.

By far the most common cause is degenerative changes affecting the cervical and lumbar regions.

Clinical features
Clinical features include:
- Pain—severe, sharp, shooting and/or burning pain radiating into the cutaneous distribution (dermatome) or muscle group (myotome) supplied by the root. It may be aggravated by movement, straining, or coughing.
- Neurologic signs—lower motor neuron signs (i.e., wasting with or without fasciculations, weakness, and reduced reflexes) in the affected myotome and sensory impairment in the affected dermatome.

Specific radiculopathies
Lateral cervical disc protrusion
Lateral disc protrusion in the cervical region (Fig. 27.2) often causes severe pain in the upper limb. A disc protrusion at C7 is the most common lesion. Root pain radiates into the affected myotome (scapula, triceps, and forearm extensors in a C7 root lesion) and a sensory disturbance (paresthesias and numbness) in the affected dermatome.

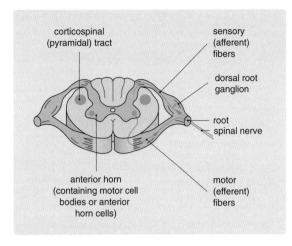

Fig. 27.1 Anatomy of spinal roots.

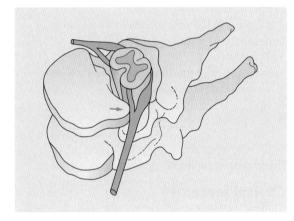

Fig. 27.2 Lateral disc protrusion in the cervical region.

Subsequently, there is wasting and weakness of the muscles innervated by the root (triceps and wrist and finger extensors in a C7 lesion), and the reflexes involved in this root will be lost (triceps jerk in a C7 lesion).

Lesions can be visualized on magnetic resonance imaging (MRI) or myelography with computed tomography (CT). When only pain is present, most cases recover with rest, with the aid of a neck collar, and analgesia. When recovery is delayed, especially if neurologic signs exist, surgical root decompression may be performed.

Lateral lumbar disc protrusion
The most common lesion in the lumbar region causes compression of L5 and S1 roots due to lateral

prolapse of L4/L5 and L5/S1 discs, respectively. This results in low back pain and "sciatica" (pain radiating down the buttock and posterior lower limb). The onset may be acute or subacute.

There is limitation of straight-leg raising in the affected leg. There may be weakness of extension of the great toe (L5) or of plantar flexion (S1). The reflexes may be lost (ankle jerk in an S1 root lesion, or, rarely, the knee jerk in an L3/L4 lesion). Sensory loss may be found in the affected dermatome.

Investigations include plain x-ray, MRI, and myelography. Most cases resolve with rest and analgesia, but decompressive surgery may be required.

Central lumbar disc protrusion (cauda equina syndrome)
Since the spinal cord ends at L1, a central disc protrusion below this level will result in a radiculopathy. As multiple nerve roots (cauda equina) are involved, such a lesion will produce back pain, lower motor neuron weakness of the legs and feet, sacral numbness, retention of urine, bowel dysfunction, and impotence.

The onset may be acute, causing a flaccid paraparesis, or may be chronic, producing a picture identical to intermittent claudication caused by vascular insufficiency. A patient with back pain who develops retention of urine should be suspected of having a central lumbar disc protrusion. Urgent imaging and decompression should follow.

Plexopathies (lesions of the brachial or lumbosacral plexus)

Causes
Causes of plexopathies include:
- Trauma.
- Neuralgic amyotrophy.
- Malignant infiltration.
- Compression.
- Thoracic outlet syndrome (cervical rib).

Trauma is the most common cause of a brachial plexus lesion, and early referral to a specialist unit with experience in the surgical repair of plexus injuries is advised.

Clinical features

The clinical features depend on the affected regions of the plexus.

Brachial plexus

Upper plexus lesion (C5–C6)

An upper plexus lesion may be caused by traction on the arm at birth (Erb–Duchenne paralysis) or by falling on the shoulder. It causes weakness and wasting of:

- Deltoid.
- Supraspinatus and infraspinatus.
- Biceps.
- Brachioradialis.

There may be mild weakness of shoulder adduction, and if the damage is proximal, the nerve to rhomboids and the long thoracic nerve may be involved. There will be loss of the biceps jerk and sensory impairment in the C5–C6 dermatomes.

Posterior cord lesion (C5–C8)

A posterior cord lesion causes weakness and wasting of:

- Deltoid.
- Triceps.
- Wrist extensors (extensor carpi radialis longus and brevis, and extensor carpi ulnaris).
- Extensor digitorum.

There will be loss of the triceps jerk and sensory impairment in the affected dermatomes.

Lower plexus lesion (C8, T1)

A lower plexus lesion may be caused by forced abduction of the arm at birth (Klumpke's paralysis), trauma, or lesions pushing from below (e.g., cervical rib, Pancoast tumor).

This results in paralysis of the intrinsic hand muscles, producing a claw hand; C8, T1 sensory loss; and a Horner's syndrome (miosis, ptosis, and enophthalmos) if the T1 root is involved.

Lumbosacral plexus

Symptoms of a lumbosacral plexus lesion may be unilateral or bilateral depending upon causation. Most common are diabetic proximal neuropathy ("amyotrophy") and malignant infiltration in the pelvis. Weakness, reflex change, and sensory loss are dependent on the location and extent of plexus damage. In general, the following features are found:

- Upper plexus lesion—weakness of hip flexion and adduction, with anterior leg sensory loss.
- Lower plexus lesion—weakness of the posterior thigh (hamstrings) and foot muscles, with posterior leg sensory loss.

Specific plexopathies

Neuralgic amyotrophy (brachial neuritis)

Neuralgic amyotrophy is a condition in which severe pain in the muscles of the shoulder is followed 2–7 days later, as the pain lessens, by rapid wasting and weakness in various muscles of the arm, usually proximal ones. Reflex loss occurs. Sensory findings are usually minor. It is thought to be inflammatory in nature and may follow viral infection or vaccination. Recovery is gradual over many months but may not be complete. Recurrent episodes can occur.

Neuralgic amyotrophy may be part of hereditary liability to pressure palsies (HLPP), which is associated with a deletion on chromosome 17. There may be evidence of a diffuse neuropathy on nerve conduction studies.

Diabetic amyotrophy

Diabetic amyotrophy, which involves the lumbar plexus, is usually seen in older men with diabetes and is associated with periods of poor glycemic control. Presentation is with painful wasting, usually strikingly asymmetrical, of the quadriceps muscles. There is loss of the knee jerks and extreme tenderness in the affected area. This is resolved with careful control of blood glucose.

Cervical rib (thoracic outlet syndrome)

In thoracic outlet syndrome, a fibrous band or cervical rib extending from the tip of the transverse process of C7 to the first rib stretches the lower part of the brachial plexus (C8, T1). There is pain along the ulnar border of the forearm, and sensory loss initially in the distribution of T1, with wasting of the thenar muscles predominantly. There may also be a Horner's syndrome.

Some patients develop a vascular syndrome with compression of the subclavian artery or vein. The vascular and neurological syndromes rarely coexist. Treatment is surgical.

Pancoast tumor

There can be involvement of the brachial plexus by an apical lung tumor (usually squamous cell carcinoma) affecting C8, T1-derived roots.

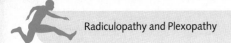

Clinically, there is:
- Severe pain.
- Ipsilateral weak and wasted hand.
- Sensory loss (C8, T1).
- Horner's syndrome

Malignant infiltration

Pelvic tumors (e.g., prostate, cervix) can infiltrate or metastasize to the lumbosacral plexus. This is usually associated with severe pain.

28. Disorders of Peripheral Nerve

Anatomy

Peripheral nerves are made up of numerous axons bound together by three types of connective tissue—endoneurium, perineurium, and epineurium (Fig. 28.1). The vasa nervorum located in the epineurium provides the blood supply.

Peripheral nerve trunks contain myelinated and unmyelinated fibers. Myelin is a protein–lipid complex that forms an insulating layer around some axons, resulting in increased rates of conduction in these fibers.

All axons have a cellular sheath, the Schwann cell, but only in some does the membrane of the cell "spiral" around the axon, forming the multilayered myelin sheath.

Schwann cells of myelinated nerves are separated by nodes of Ranvier—at these points, the axons are bare. During conduction, impulses jump from one node to the next, which is called saltatory conduction.

Conduction in unmyelinated nerves is slower and dependent on the diameter of the axon.

Nerve fiber type

Within the peripheral nerve, the axons vary structurally and this is related to function. Three distinct types of fiber can be distinguished (Fig. 28.2). All are myelinated apart from the C fibers, which carry impulses from painful stimuli.

Pathologic processes

The function of peripheral nerves can be disrupted by damage to the cell body, the axon, the myelin sheath, the connective tissue, or the blood supply.

Two basic pathologic processes occur:
- Wallerian degeneration: the axon degenerates distally, following section or severe injury, with degeneration of the myelin. The process occurs within 7–10 days of injury and this portion of the nerve is inexcitable electrically. Regeneration can occur since the basement membrane of the Schwann cell survives and acts as a skeleton along which the axon regrows up to a rate of about 1 mm per day.
- Demyelination: segmental destruction of the myelin sheath occurs without axonal damage. The primary lesion affects the Schwann cell and causes marked slowing of conduction or conduction block. Local demyelination is caused by pressure (e.g., entrapment neuropathies) or by inflammation (e.g., Guillain Barré syndrome).

Definitions of neuropathies

A neuropathy is a pathologic process that affects a peripheral nerve or nerves and may involve axonal degeneration (Wallerian degeneration) or demyelination, as discussed above.

In *mononeuropathy* a single nerve is affected. If multiple single nerves are affected in an asymmetrical pattern, it is termed multifocal neuropathy or *mononeuritis multiplex*.

Polyneuropathy is a diffuse, symmetrical disease process that is usually distal with some proximal progression. It can be acute, subacute, or chronic. It may be progressive, relapsing, or transient and can be motor, sensory, autonomic, or mixed (sensorimotor with or without autonomic).

Symptoms of peripheral nerve disease

Sensory symptoms
Negative symptoms (loss of sensation)
Large myelinated fiber disease causes loss of touch and joint-position sense (proprioception), leading to:

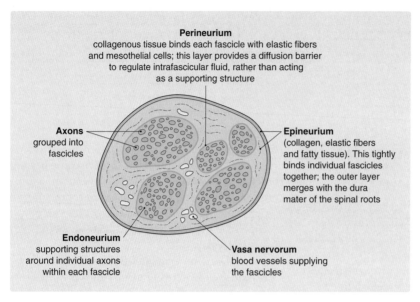

Perineurium
collagenous tissue binds each fascicle with elastic fibers and mesothelial cells; this layer provides a diffusion barrier to regulate intrafascicular fluid, rather than acting as a supporting structure

Axons
grouped into fascicles

Epineurium
(collagen, elastic fibers and fatty tissue). This tightly binds individual fascicles together; the outer layer merges with the dura mater of the spinal roots

Endoneurium
supporting structures around individual axons within each fascicle

Vasa nervorum
blood vessels supplying the fascicles

Fig. 28.1 Transverse section of a peripheral nerve.

Fiber types in peripheral nerve			
Fiber type	**Fiber diameter (µm)**	**Velocity (m/s)**	**Function/nerve type**
Type A (myelinated): group I	12–20	90	vibration and position sense alpha motor neurons
group II	6–12	50	touch and pressure afferents
group III	1–6	30	gamma afferents
Type B (myelinated)	2–6	10	autonomic preganglionic
Type C (unmyelinated)	<1	2	pain and temperature afferents autonomic postganglionic

Fig. 28.2 Fiber types in peripheral nerve.

- Difficulty discriminating textures.
- Feet and hands feeling like "cotton wool."
- Gait unsteady through loss of position sense, especially at night when vision cannot compensate.

Small unmyelinated fiber disease causes loss of pain and temperature appreciation, leading to:
- Painless burns and trauma.
- Damage to joints (Charcot's joint), resulting in painless deformity.

Positive symptoms
Large myelinated fiber disease can cause paresthesias ("pins and needles").

Small unmyelinated fiber disease produces painful positive symptoms:
- Burning sensations.
- Dysesthesia—pain on gentle touch.
- Hyperalgesia—lowered threshold to pain.
- Hyperpathia—pain threshold is elevated, but pain is excessively felt.

- Lightening pains—sudden, very severe, shooting pains, which usually suggest a diagnosis of tabes dorsalis (late syphilis).

Motor symptoms

Weakness is usually the main presenting feature. This is usually distal (e.g., difficulty clearing the curb when walking or weak hands), but in some neuropathies can be proximal (e.g., difficulty climbing stairs or combing hair).

Patients may also complain of cramps and twitching of muscles (fasciculations), although these symptoms are more commonly due to neuronopathies (diseases affecting the anterior horn cell, e.g. motor neuron disease).

Signs of peripheral neuropathy

Sensory examination

Functions of large myelinated sensory fibers include:

- Light touch.
- Two-point discrimination.
- Vibration sense.
- Joint-position sense.

Functions of small unmyelinated and thinly myelinated sensory fibers include:

- Temperature perception.
- Pain perception.

A classic polyneuropathy will produce sensory loss in the characteristic "glove-and-stocking" distribution. This phenomenon is usually length related; therefore, signs in the hands will not develop until there is sensory loss up to at least mid-shin level.

When joint-position sense is lost, gait is abnormal ("sensory ataxia"). Romberg's test is positive (loss of joint-position sense is compensated for by vision, therefore when the eyes are closed, the stance becomes unsteady, whereas it is steady when the eyes are open).

Sensory examination should include the search for neuropathic burns, trauma, and Charcot joints.

Motor examination

The classic features of a lower motor neuron abnormality include:

- Distal wasting of muscles—wasting can occur with generalized weight loss, but weakness is rare; however, the muscles may fatigue easily in this context.
- Weakness of muscles.
- Depressed or absent tendon reflexes.
- Fasciculations.

Investigation of peripheral neuropathy

In up to 30% of cases, the cause of a neuropathy may not be identified. The following investigations help in the diagnosis:

- Blood tests—routine blood tests to exclude certain causes of peripheral neuropathy should include complete blood count (CBC), erythrocyte sedimentation rate (ESR), C-reactive protein (CRP), urea and electrolytes (especially renal function tests), liver function tests, glucose, hemoglobin A1C, thyroid function, vitamin B_{12}, and protein electrophoresis.
- Nerve conduction studies—these can differentiate axonal degeneration (reduced amplitude) from demyelination (reduced conduction velocity) and can characterize whether sensory and/or motor fibers are involved. They can also localize the sites of abnormality (e.g., in entrapment neuropathies).
- Electromyography (EMG)—use of a fine needle inserted into the muscle can discern whether complete or partial denervation is present and whether reinnervation is occurring. This can help in localization depending on the distribution of muscles affected.
- Nerve biopsy—the sural nerve is the one most commonly biopsied provided that its conduction is abnormal. Using light and electron microscopy, further pathological information can be gleaned.
- Cerebrospinal fluid (CSF) examination—this may be helpful, for example, in inflammatory demyelinating neuropathies (Guillain Barré syndrome or chronic inflammatory demyelinating polyradiculoneuropathy—see pp. 169–170), when the protein content is usually raised.

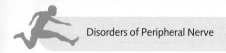

Specific neuropathies

Mononeuropathies
Peripheral nerve compression and entrapment neuropathies

Nerves can be damaged by compression either acutely (e.g., by pressure during an operating room procedure) or chronically (e.g., entrapment neuropathy). This usually causes localized demyelination, although, if prolonged, it may lead to axonal degeneration.

Acute compression occurs in nerves that lie superficially (e.g., the common peroneal nerve at the fibular head, caused by prolonged knee crossing, or the radial nerve as it passes round the humerus, causing "Saturday-night palsy").

Entrapment occurs when the nerve passes through tight anatomic spaces (e.g., carpal tunnel syndrome).

The most common of these conditions are presented below.

Carpal tunnel syndrome (median nerve compression at the wrist)

Carpal tunnel syndrome is usually idiopathic but can be associated with:

- Hypothyroidism.
- Pregnancy.
- Diabetes mellitus.
- Rheumatoid arthritis.
- Acromegaly.

It presents with tingling, pain, and numbness in the hand, especially first thing in the morning and, in some cases, with weakness of the thenar muscles. Sensory loss of the palm and the radial three-and-a-half fingers develops and there is wasting of abductor pollicis brevis. Tinel's sign may be present—tapping on the carpal tunnel reproduces tingling and pain. Diagnosis is by electrophysiology. Surgical decompression is the definitive procedure, although splints and steroid injections may provide temporary relief.

Ulnar nerve compression

Ulnar nerve compression is less common than carpal tunnel syndrome. Entrapment typically occurs at the elbow, where the nerve is compressed within the cubital tunnel. It can follow fracture of the ulna or prolonged or recurrent pressure at this site.

There is wasting and weakness of ulnar-innervated muscles and sensory loss in the ulnar one-and-a-half fingers.

Electrophysiology localizes the lesion. Surgical decompression or transposition of the nerve may be necessary.

A further ulnar compression neuropathy can occur in the deep, motor branch as it passes across the palm. This is due to regular pressure from tools (e.g., screwdrivers), crutches, or handlebars.

Radial nerve compression

Radial nerve compression occurs when the radial nerve is compressed against the humerus (e.g., when the arm is draped over the back of a chair for several hours ["Saturday-night palsy"]) and results in wristdrop and weakness of finger extension and brachioradialis. Recovery is usually spontaneous but may take up to 3 months.

Common peroneal nerve palsy

Common peroneal nerve palsy occurs when the common peroneal nerve is compressed at the fibular head and can result from prolonged squatting or leg crossing, wearing a tight plaster cast, prolonged bed rest, or coma. It results in a footdrop and weakness of eversion, with sensory loss on the anterolateral border of the shin and dorsum of the foot. Recovery is usual, but not invariable, within a few months.

Meralgia paraesthetica

Entrapment of the lateral femoral cutaneous nerve of the thigh, beneath the inguinal ligament, causes burning, tingling, and numbness on the anterolateral surface of the thigh. It usually occurs in overweight patients and weight loss may help.

Multifocal neuropathy (mononeuritis multiplex)

Certain systemic illnesses are associated with multiple mononeuropathies. These include:

- Diabetes mellitus.
- Connective tissue disease (e.g., polyarteritis nodosa, systemic lupus erythematosus [SLE], rheumatoid arthritis).
- Sarcoidosis.
- Malignancy.
- Amyloidosis.
- Neurofibromatosis.
- AIDS.
- Leprosy.

Polyneuropathies

Polyneuropathies can be classified according to their mode of onset, functional or pathologic type, distribution, or causation. The classification used below is based on causation.

Hereditary neuropathies

This section will consider the group of conditions known as the hereditary motor sensory neuropathies (HMSN). These are also Charcot–Marie–Tooth disease. Other types of hereditary neuropathy will be considered in Chapter 37.

With the advent of molecular genetic studies, the original classification system for HMSN is undergoing modification. Categories are as follows:

- HMSN type I (most common form)—demyelinating neuropathy with hypertrophy ("onion-bulb" formation).
- HMSN type II—axonal neuropathy.
- HMSN type III (Dejerine–Sottas disease)—demyelination with gross hypertrophy; often the CSF protein is raised due to hypertrophied nerve roots.
- Complex forms of HMSN—additional features such as optic atrophy, retinitis pigmentosa, deafness, and spastic paraparesis can coexist.
- Distal spinal muscular atrophy (distal SMA; spinal form of Charcot–Marie–Tooth disease)—historical terminology includes this condition in the classification. It is actually a disease of the anterior horn cell and not the peripheral nerve but can produce a similar clinical picture to HMSN.

General characteristics of hereditary motor sensory neuropathies

All forms of HMSN are characterized by distal wasting of the lower limbs, which progresses, often over many years, and may involve the upper limbs.

Once the wasting in the legs is severe, they resemble "inverted champagne bottles" (Fig. 28.3). The wasting is accompanied by reduced or absent reflexes and a variable loss of sensation.

Pes cavus with clawing of the toes is almost invariable. These features may be the only signs in mild cases. Clawing of the hands may also be seen.

The age of onset varies from childhood to middle age. There is variability within subgroups and within families.

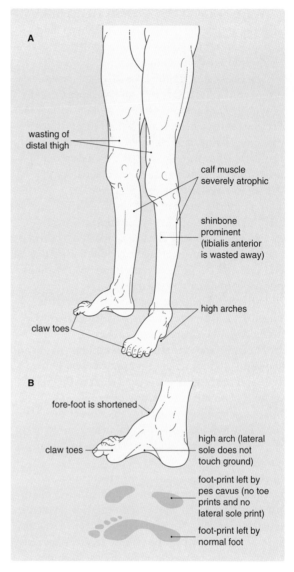

Fig. 28.3 "Inverted-champagne-bottle" legs of hereditary motor sensory neuropathy.

Inflammatory demyelinating neuropathies

The group of inflammatory demyelinating neuropathies includes an acute neuropathy (Guillain Barré syndrome [GBS]) and a chronic inflammatory demyelinating polyradiculoneuropathy (CIDP).

Guillain Barré syndrome (postinfective polyneuropathy)

GBS is an inflammatory demyelinating polyradiculoneuropathy occurring worldwide with an annual rate of 1.5 cases per 100,000 persons.

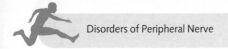

It often follows 1–3 weeks after a respiratory infection or diarrhea, which may have been mild. *Campylobacter jejuni* has been particularly implicated as a cause of the diarrhea.

The classic presentation is with distal paresthesias, often with little sensory loss, and weakness, usually proximal. The symptoms ascend over days to weeks. Facial weakness is present in 50% of cases. In severe cases, respiratory and bulbar involvement occurs, and ventilation may be required. (If the vital capacity drops to 1 or below, ventilation is mandatory.) Autonomic dysfunction may also occur.

A proximal variant of GBS involves ocular muscles and ataxia (Miller–Fisher syndrome).

Diagnosis is usually clinical, supported by slowed conduction velocities on nerve conduction studies and a raised CSF protein. Both these investigations may be normal early in the disease.

Differential diagnoses include other paralytic illnesses such as poliomyelitis, Myasthenia Gravis, botulism, and primary muscle disease.

The use of intravenous immunoglobulin has been shown to produce significant improvement in the course of the disease and is equivalent to the more invasive plasmapheresis. Corticosteroids and immunosuppressive agents have not been successful in acute GBS. Careful management of the paralyzed patient and ventilation as indicated are also essential.

Recovery, though gradual over many months, is usual but may be incomplete. Approximately 5% of patients develop a relapsing and remitting disease. A mortality rate of 10% reflects inadequate ventilatory support. By definition, the symptoms and signs cease to progress after 6 weeks or the disease becomes termed CIDP.

Chronic inflammatory demyelinating polyradiculoneuropathy

CIDP represents an often milder syndrome related to GBS but with a more protracted clinical course. The clinical and diagnostic features and pathology are similar to those of GBS. It is rarely associated with preceding infection.

The treatment of choice is corticosteroids with or without other immunosuppressive agents such as azathioprine or cyclophosphamide. Immunoglobulin and plasmapheresis can be helpful, but repeated courses are required.

Neuropathies associated with systemic disease

The peripheral nerve can be affected by a wide range of systemic diseases. The following represent a small selection of the commonest conditions.

Diabetic neuropathy

The neuropathies found in diabetes mellitus are often related to poor glycemic control. The exact cause of the nerve damage is uncertain but may relate to sorbitol accumulation or to vascular disease in both large and small vessels.

A number of different types of neuropathy complicate diabetes:

- Distal symmetrical polyneuropathy—most commonly sensory, but may be motor or autonomic.
- Proximal lower extremity asymmetrical motor neuropathy—known as diabetic amyotrophy.
- Autonomic neuropathy—with gastroparesis and resultant diarrhea, arrhythmias, and postural hypotension.
- Mononeuropathies can be single or multiple: cranial nerve lesion (especially isolated third and sixth nerve palsies), isolated peripheral nerve lesion (especially entrapment neuropathies), and mononeuritis multiplex.

Renal disease

Chronic renal failure produces a progressive sensorimotor neuropathy. The response to dialysis is variable, but the neuropathy usually improves after renal transplantation.

Carcinomatous polyneuropathy

Malignant disease, especially small-cell carcinoma of the bronchus, often produces a sensory or a sensorimotor neuropathy. The neuropathy may predate the appearance of the malignancy by months or years.

Antineuronal antibodies (anti-Hu) may be present in patients with small-cell carcinomas, which can aid diagnosis.

Hematologic malignancies such as multiple myeloma and other monoclonal gammopathies characteristically produce peripheral neuropathies.

Connective tissue diseases and vasculitides

Connective tissue diseases and vasculitides classically produce a mononeuritis multiplex, although individual diseases may produce a symmetrical sensorimotor neuropathy (especially SLE), entrapment neuropathy (rheumatoid arthritis), or trigeminal neuralgia (Sjögren's syndrome).

Porphyria

Acute intermittent porphyria produces a predominantly motor neuropathy in addition to abdominal pain, psychosis, and seizures.

Amyloidosis

In amyloidosis, amyloid is deposited around the vessels in the nerve, causing distortion. The neuropathy is characterized by predominantly sensory, painful, dysesthetic features. Autonomic features are common.

Alcoholic neuropathy

Alcoholic neuropathy is one of the most common forms of peripheral neuropathy (up to 30% of all cases of neuropathy).

It progresses slowly, with distal sensory loss, paresthesias, and burning pains. Distal muscle weakness may occur and spread proximally, with muscle cramps and gait disturbance.

Whether the neuropathy is caused primarily by the alcohol is clouded by the fact that many alcoholics are deficient, particularly in thiamine and other B vitamins, as well as often having an inadequate general dietary intake.

Abstinence from alcohol, supplementation of thiamine, and a balanced diet constitute the main therapy. The painful symptoms may be controlled with the use of carbamazepine, gabapentin, or tricyclic antidepressants.

Neuropathies caused by nutritional deficiencies

A number of vitamin deficiencies can result in neuropathy.

Thiamine (vitamin B$_1$) deficiency (beriberi)

Thiamine deficiency is highly implicated in the causation of alcoholic neuropathy. In addition to the peripheral neuropathy, deficiency can cause Wernicke–Korsakoff syndrome (see Chapter 36).

Pyridoxine (vitamin B$_6$) deficiency

Pyridoxine deficiency causes a mainly sensory neuropathy. It may be precipitated by isoniazid therapy for TB, and pyridoxine is therefore given in association with this drug.

Vitamin B$_{12}$ deficiency (subacute combined degeneration of the cord)

Peripheral neuropathy occurs as part of subacute combined degeneration of the cord, with spastic paraparesis, loss of proprioception, paresthesias, and, in some cases, slowly progressive dementia. Treatment involves intramuscular replacement injections (see Chapter 25).

Vitamin E deficiency

Vitamin E deficiency occurs in the context of fat malabsorption. The onset of neurologic symptoms takes many years. It involves a large-fiber sensory neuropathy with spinocerebellar degeneration.

Neuropathies caused by drugs and toxins

Drugs

A wide variety of drugs are known to cause a peripheral neuropathy. Most produce a chronic, progressive, sensorimotor polyneuropathy and are generally reversible. Examples of the most common include:

- Sensory axonal neuropathy—chloramphenicol, isoniazid (by affecting pyridoxine metabolism), phenytoin.
- Motor axonal neuropathy—amphotericin, dapsone, gold.
- Sensorimotor axonal neuropathy—chlorambucil, cisplatin, disulfiram, nitrofurantoin, vincristine.
- Sensorimotor demyelinating neuropathy— amiodarone.

Toxins

A wide variety of metals and industrial toxins have been shown to cause polyneuropathy. Peripheral nerve involvement is often accompanied by other systemic features. For example:

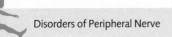
- Lead causes a motor neuropathy.
- Arsenic and thallium cause a painful peripheral sensory neuropathy.
- Acrylamide, trichloroethylene, and fat-soluble hydrocarbons (e.g., as in glue sniffing) cause a progressive polyneuropathy.

Summary

The causes of peripheral neuropathies are summarized in Fig. 28.4.

Causes of peripheral neuropathies	

inflammatory	Guillain Barré syndrome
	chronic inflammatory
	   demyelinating
	     polyradiculoneuropathy

metabolic	diabetes renal disease porphyria
nutritional deficiencies	vitamin B_1 vitamin B_6 vitamin B_{12} vitamin E
toxic	drugs alcohol lead arsenic
connective tissue disease	systemic lupus erythematosus rheumatoid arthritis polyarteritis
malignancy	bronchus breast myeloma
hereditary	HMSN syndromes
trauma	entrapment mononeuropathies limb injuries

Fig. 28.4 Summary of causes of peripheral neuropathies.

29. Disorders of Neuromuscular Transmission

Normal anatomy and physiology

The normal anatomy and physiology of the neuromuscular junction are outlined in Fig. 29.1. In motor nerves, when the stimulus reaches the end of the nerve terminal, acetylcholine is released from vesicles via voltage-gated calcium channels. The acetylcholine crosses the synaptic cleft and binds to acetylcholine receptors on the postsynaptic muscle end-plate membrane. This results in depolarization and subsequent contraction of the muscle. The acetylcholine is then broken down by acetylcholinesterase, which is bound to the basal lamina in the synaptic folds.

Two main diseases of neuromuscular transmission will be discussed in this chapter—Myasthenia Gravis and Lambert–Eaton myasthenic syndrome (LEMS).

Myasthenia Gravis

Myasthenia Gravis is an acquired immunologic disorder of unknown cause, in which antibodies are directed against the postsynaptic acetylcholine receptor. This results in weakness and fatiguability of skeletal muscle groups. The most commonly affected muscles are the proximal limb, ocular, and bulbar muscles.

There is an associated abnormality of the thymus in patients with Myasthenia Gravis. Thymic hyperplasia is found in 70% of patients below the age of 40 years. In 10% of all patients with Myasthenia Gravis, a thymic tumor (thymoma) is found, the incidence increasing with age. In patients with thymoma, antibodies to striated muscle may also be found.

Two distinct groups of patients appear to develop Myasthenia Gravis, split by age and sex:
- Young women (20–35 years), who tend to have an acute, severely fluctuating, more generalized condition, with increased association with HLA-B8 and HLA-DR3.
- Older men (60–75 years), who tend to have a more oculobulbar presentation.

There is some crossover between the groups, and Myasthenia Gravis is seen in young men and older women, but much less frequently.

Clinical features

The clinical features of Myasthenia Gravis are listed in Fig. 29.2. The most important of these is the fatiguability, causing fluctuating weakness, which is worse after exercise and, usually, at the end of the day.

Fatiguability can be demonstrated by exercising affected muscles. For example, if a patient in whom ptosis is sometimes apparent looks upward for a few seconds, the ptosis will become apparent, and the eyes may drift to the neutral position (termed the "curtain sign"). Similar maneuvers can be carried out for the proximal limb muscles.

Limb reflexes are normal or hyperactive, but fatigue on repeated testing. Muscle wasting occurs in 15% of cases. Sensory examination is normal.

Investigations
Tensilon test (edrophonium)

Edrophonium is a fast-acting anticholinesterase, i.e., it antagonizes the action of acetylcholinesterase and thus prevents the breakdown of acetylcholine, allowing it to competitively compete with acetylcholine receptor antibodies. When given as an intravenous bolus, usually with atropine to prevent cardiac side effects, weakness is improved in seconds, the effect lasting for 2–3 minutes. It acts as a diagnostic test for Myasthenia Gravis.

Serum acetylcholine receptor antibody

The highly specific acetylcholine receptor antibody is present in the serum of up to 80% of patients with generalized Myasthenia Gravis.

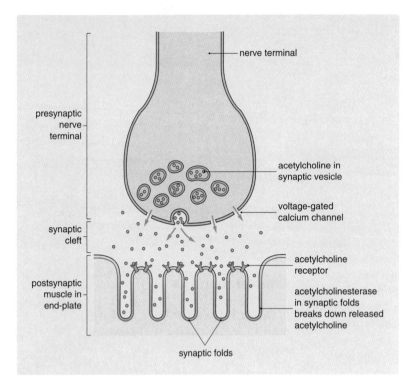

Fig. 29.1 The neuromuscular junction. Antibodies directed against acetylcholine receptors cause Myasthenia Gravis, whereas antibodies against the presynaptic voltage-gated calcium channels cause Lambert-Eaton myasthenic syndrome.

Symptoms of Myasthenia Gravis	
ocular	ptosis diplopia
other cranial muscles	weak face and jaw dysarthria dysphonia dysphagia
limb weakness	usually proximal—shoulder and hips
axial weakness	neck and trunk respiratory muscle

Fig. 29.2 Symptoms of Myasthenia Gravis.

Serum MUSK antibody

Recent reports have found circulating antibodies to muscle-specific kinase (MUSK) in 50–70% of seronegative patients. These patients tend to have more ocular-bulbar weakness.

Electromyography

There are two classic electromyographic findings in Myasthenia Gravis:

- A decrement in amplitude of the compound muscle action potential following repetitive stimulation.
- Increased jitter using a single-fiber electrode.

Thymus imaging

It is always essential to image the chest with computed tomography or magnetic resonance imaging for the presence of thymic hyperplasia or tumor, as removal of a hyperplastic thymus improves the condition in many patients.

Autoantibodies

Other autoantibodies may be present, especially those against striated muscle and thyroid.

Management

The illness may have a protracted and fluctuating course. Acute exacerbations may be unpredictable or may follow infections or treatment with certain drugs (aminoglycosides, beta blockers, calcium channel blockers, magnesium, D-penicillamine). It is important to recognize respiratory involvement, as assisted ventilation may be required. Patients may remit permanently, however, especially after thymectomy or with immunosuppressive treatment.

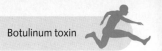

Oral acetylcholinesterases

Pyridostigmine is the most widely used drug, with a duration of action of about 3–5 hours. The patient's response will determine the dosage required.

Overdosage causes a cholinergic crisis with severe weakness, which may be difficult to differentiate from the myasthenic weakness. Colic and diarrhea may also occur.

Acetylcholinesterases are excellent symptomatic drugs but do not alter the natural history of the disease.

Thymectomy

In patients with thymic hyperplasia, thymectomy, for unknown reasons, improves the prognosis of the disease, especially in those under 40 years of age and in those who have had the disease for less than 10 years.

In patients with a thymoma, surgery is essential to remove a potentially malignant tumor, but it rarely causes improvement of the myasthenia.

Immunosuppression

Corticosteroids provide the mainstay of immunosuppressive treatment. They succeed in 70% of patients, but must be increased slowly, preferably in hospital, as there is often a temporary exacerbation of symptoms before the therapeutic effect.

Plasmapheresis is sometimes used, especially during an acute exacerbation or when there is respiratory involvement. The effects only last a few days, however.

Azathioprine is used as a steroid-sparing agent.

Lambert–Eaton myasthenic syndrome

In LEMS, a rare condition, antibodies are directed against the voltage-gated calcium channels. This results in a failure of acetylcholine release from the presynaptic nerve terminal. In many cases, it is a nonmetastatic manifestation of malignancy of a small-cell carcinoma of the lung (paraneoplastic syndrome).

It is characterized by weakness of the proximal limb muscles and occasionally ptosis, but other cranial nerves are typically spared. There may be fatiguability, but characteristically there is a paradoxical improvement in power after exercise. Reflexes are usually absent, but these may return following exercise.

The diagnosis can be confirmed electromyographically by an "increment" of the compound muscle action potential after repetitive stimulation (the opposite to Myasthenia Gravis). A search should be made for malignancy, especially bronchial.

Guanethidine hydrochloride and 4-aminopyridine may enhance acetylcholine release. Steroids and plasmapheresis may also help.

Other myasthenic syndromes

Rarer myasthenic syndromes include:
- Congenital Myasthenia Gravis.
- Neonatal Myasthenia Gravis.
- Penicillamine-induced myasthenia.

Botulinum toxin

Infective botulism (a form of food poisoning—*Clostridium botulinum*), a very rare condition, resembles severe, acute Myasthenia Gravis. However, this very powerful neuromuscular-blocking toxin is used routinely in neurologic practice, in small doses, to treat unwanted muscular activity. The indications include cervical dystonia, blepharospasm, and severe limb spasticity.

30. Disorders of Skeletal Muscle

Anatomy

Skeletal muscle is made up of large numbers of multinucleated muscle fibers, which have an outer membrane (sarcolemma) and cytoplasm (sarcoplasm) and in which lie the contractile components of the muscle (myofibrils). The fibers are separated by connective tissue (endomysium) and arranged in bundles (fasciculi). Each fasciculus has a connective tissue sheath (perimysium). The muscle is made up of a number of fasciculi bound together and surrounded by a connective tissue sheath (epimysium) (Fig. 30.1).

There are two broad types of muscle fiber, which are functionally different:

- Type I—rich in myoglobulin, with low metabolism (aerobic), and rich in sarcoplasm (slow twitch, red).
- Type II—low in myoglobulin, with high metabolism (aerobic or anaerobic) and little sarcoplasm (fast twitch, white).

Clinical features of muscle disease

Muscle has rather uniform structure and function; thus diseases of muscles from a variety of causes can produce similar clinical features.

Weakness

Weakness of muscles is a characteristic finding in myopathies. Each muscle disease exhibits a particular pattern of involvement (e.g., proximal limb, facial, and proximal upper arm), which is an important diagnostic clue. Careful examination of all muscle groups is important to classify a myopathy, and to differentiate it from a neuropathy or central nervous system (CNS) disorder.

Changes in muscle contractility

Myotonia—persistence of contraction, often for several seconds, during attempted relaxation—is found in myotonic dystrophy, paramyotonia congenita, hyperkalemic periodic paralysis, and congenital myotonia. On electromyography (EMG), the characteristic findings consist of rhythmic discharges. This phenomenon may also be elicited by a sharp tap on the muscle belly (percussion myotonia). Myotonia must be differentiated from neuromyotonia, which is derived from nerve abnormality.

In McArdle's syndrome, there is a characteristic fixed shortening of the muscle that follows a series of strong contractions, especially when ischemic—true contracture. This needs to be differentiated from cramp.

Changes in muscle tone

There may be a loss of tone (hypotonia) secondary to disease of muscle.

Changes in muscle bulk

Atrophy results with muscular dystrophies or is caused by a lower motor neuron lesion.

Enlargement of muscle may be the result of overactivity or an early sign in certain dystrophies, caused by infiltration of fat, exacerbating the weakness (pseudohypertrophy).

Pain

Pain is a rare complaint in primary muscle disease except in deficiencies of certain enzymes of the glycolytic or fat pathways or when the disease involves blood vessels within the muscle (e.g., polymyalgia rheumatica).

Family history

Many muscle diseases are inherited; therefore, a full family history is essential. Inherited muscles diseases include:

- X-linked—Duchenne muscular dystrophy, Becker's muscular dystrophy, Emery–Dreifuss dystrophy.

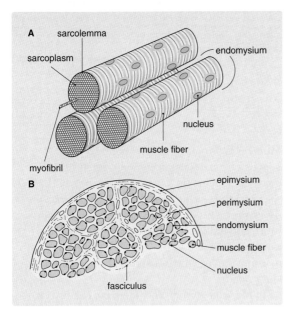

Fig. 30.1 Normal skeletal muscle morphology: (A) longitudinal muscle fibers; (B) cross-section of muscle.

Hereditary and acquired myopathies		
Hereditary myopathies	muscular dystrophies	Duchenne Becker's facioscapulohumeral limb-girdle
	myotonic disorders	myotonic dystrophy myotonia congenita
	metabolic myopathies	myophosphorylase deficiency (McArdle's disease) phosphofructokinase deficiency lactate dehydrogenase deficiency carnitine palmityl transferase deficiency
	periodic paralyses	hypokalemic hyperkalemic
	mitochondrial myopathies	Keam Sayres
Acquired myopathies	inflammatory myopathies	polymyositis dermatomyositis
	metabolic or endocrine myopathies	Cushing's syndrome thyroid disease disorders of calcium hypokalemia corticosteroids alcohol

Fig. 30.2 Hereditary and acquired myopathies.

- Autosomal dominant—facioscapulohumeral dystrophy, scapuloperoneal dystrophy, myotonic dystrophy.
- Autosomal recessive—limb-girdle dystrophy, all deficiencies of enzymes of glycolytic and lipid metabolism.
- Mitochondrial—Kearn–Sayres syndrome.

Investigation of muscle disease

The diagnosis may be possible from the clinical features in some causes of muscle disease. Additionally, helpful tests include:
- Serum creatine phosphokinase (CPK), creatine kinase (CK)—often highly raised in many dystrophies and in inflammatory muscle disorders (e.g., polymyositis).
- EMG—needle examination will reveal "myopathic units" (small, short-duration, spiky polyphasic units). There may be evidence of myotonic discharges in myotonias.
- Muscle biopsy—this can yield information about fiber type (type I or II), inflammation, and dystrophic and histochemical changes. Electron microscopy is sometimes required.

Specific muscle diseases

Myopathies can be subdivided as in Fig. 30.2. Important examples are further discussed below.

Hereditary myopathies
Muscular dystrophies
Duchenne muscular dystrophy
Duchenne muscular dystrophy is an X-linked recessive condition caused by an absence of dystrophin, occurring in 20–30/100,000 liveborn males. It affects skeletal and cardiac muscle.

With Duchenne muscular dystrophy, there is no abnormality at birth, but the condition is apparent by the fourth year. The boy is usually wheelchair-bound by 10 years old, and death is usual by the age of 20, from respiratory failure or cardiomyopathy.

There is initially proximal muscle weakness with pseudohypertrophy of the calves. The weakness then spreads. When rising to an erect position, there is a characteristic maneuver in which the patient has to "climb" his legs with his hands (Gower's sign) (Fig. 30.3).

The diagnosis of Duchenne muscular dystrophy is often made clinically. However, the CK is grossly elevated (often >10,000 U/L). The EMG is myopathic, and muscle biopsy shows fatty infiltration and absence of staining for dystrophin.

There is no cure for Duchenne muscular dystrophy, so the management is supportive. Steroids may provide short-term improvement. Genetic counseling is important—in carrier females, the CK is often raised and the EMG may be myopathic, although there are no clinical signs. There is also an accurate and rapid DNA probe available, so accurate carrier and prenatal diagnosis can be made.

Becker's muscular dystrophy

Becker's muscular dystrophy is also an X-linked recessive condition, with similar characteristics to Duchenne muscular dystrophy, but it has a much milder course. Dystrophin is altered rather than absent.

The symptoms of Becker's muscular dystrophy begin in the first decade, although often they are not noticed until later. Boys continue to walk into their teens and early adult life. Cramps associated with exercise are common. Cardiomyopathy can be worse than the weakness.

Other muscular dystrophies

Other muscular dystrophies include facioscapulohumeral dystrophy (autosomal dominant), scapuloperoneal dystrophy (autosomal dominant), and limb-girdle dystrophy (mixed inheritance, can be autosomal recessive). The patterns of weakness are described in their names. The clinical presentations vary from mild and slowly progressive to rapidly fatal.

Myotonic disorders
Myotonic dystrophy (dystrophia myotonica)

Myotonic dystrophy is an inherited condition caused by an expanded trinucleotide repeat (GTC) on chromosome 19 and thus causes "anticipation," whereby successive generations are more severely affected. The features may be very mild in some cases.

It is a multisystem disease resulting in (Fig. 30.4):

- Progressive distal muscle weakness, which may progress proximally.
- Myotonia (worse in the cold).
- Myopathic facies (weakness and thinning of the face and sternomastoids).
- Ptosis.
- Cataracts.
- Frontal balding.
- Mild intellectual impairment.
- Cardiomyopathy and conduction defects.
- Gynecomastia and testicular atrophy.
- Bronchiectasis.
- Glucose intolerance

The features develop between the ages of 20 and 50 years and progress gradually.

Metabolic myopathies

Any disturbance of the biochemical pathways that support ATP levels in muscle will cause exercise intolerance, with pain during exercise and extreme fatigue. Continued exercise will lead to destruction of muscle (rhabdomyolysis) and the release of myoglobin, which may cause renal failure.

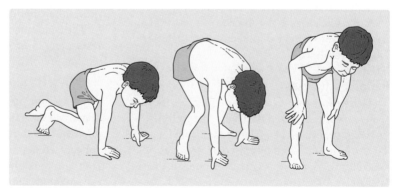

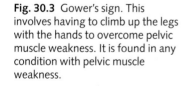

Fig. 30.3 Gower's sign. This involves having to climb up the legs with the hands to overcome pelvic muscle weakness. It is found in any condition with pelvic muscle weakness.

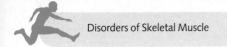

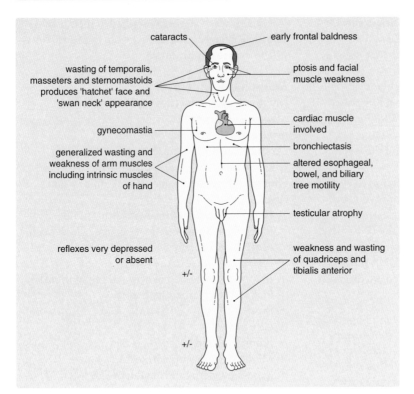

Fig. 30.4 Clinical features of myotonic dystrophy.

There are a large number of specific enzyme deficiencies, inherited via autosomal recessive genes. Only one will be discussed.

Myophosphorylase deficiency (McArdle's syndrome)

McArdle's syndrome is an autosomal recessive condition with deficiency of myophosphorylase in skeletal muscle. Symptoms begin during teenage years, with fatigue and severe pain during exercise. Continued exercises cause true contractures, which are silent on EMG (as opposed to cramp), and there is a risk of developing myoglobinuria.

A diagnostic sign is the absence of a rise in venous lactate during an ischemic exercise test (using a blood-pressure cuff).

Periodic paralyses

The periodic paralyses are rare membrane disorders that are now recognized to be among a group of disorders known as skeletal muscle channelopathies. They are characterized by episodes of sudden weakness with alterations in serum potassium levels.

Hypokalemic periodic paralysis

Hypokalemic periodic paralysis is an autosomal dominant condition that results in abnormalities of L-type calcium channels.

It becomes apparent between 10 and 20 years of age and may remit after 35 years of age. Attacks of generalized weakness develop after a heavy carbohydrate meal or after a period of rest following strenuous exertion (e.g., the following morning).

During an attack, the serum potassium falls to below 3.0 mmol/L. Attacks may last from 4 to 24 hours. The weakness responds to treatment with potassium chloride.

The condition is rarely fatal, as the diaphragm and respiratory muscles tend to be spared. Similar weakness with hypokalemia may occur in thyrotoxicosis.

Hyperkalemic periodic paralysis

Hyperkalemic periodic paralysis is an autosomal dominant condition that results in abnormalities of voltage-gated sodium channels.

It becomes apparent between 5 and 15 years of age and tends to remit after 20 years of age; however, a chronic proximal myopathy may persist. The attacks of weakness, especially of proximal muscles, become apparent 30 minutes to 2 hours after exercise and during fasting.

During an attack, the serum potassium is raised above 5.0mmol/L. Attacks may be terminated by intravenous calcium gluconate. Prophylaxis with thiazide diuretics or acetazolamide can be used.

Mitochondrial myopathies

The final oxidative pathway involves the respiratory chain in mitochondria, which have their own DNA. Abnormalities of mitochondrial DNA (maternally inherited) cause a wide range of different conditions affecting muscle, the CNS, and other systems within the body.

Acquired myopathies
Inflammatory myopathies
Polymyositis and dermatomyositis

Polymyositis and dermatomyositis are conditions in which there is inflammation within the muscle. There may be associated connective tissue disease (25%) or underlying carcinoma (10%), especially if skin changes are present (dermatomyositis).

Polymyositis and dermatomyositis usually present in the fourth to fifth decade, with women more commonly affected than men. Proximal muscle weakness is the cardinal symptom (difficulty rising from a chair or climbing stairs). Pain and tenderness of the muscles occurs in less than half the patients.

The associated skin changes (dermatomyositis) include:

- Macular erythema on the face—especially in the periorbital area, where it is heliotrope (blue–violet) in color.
- Erythematous plaques over the dorsal aspects of the fingers (Gottron's papules).
- Nail-fold hemorrhages.
- Photosensitivity.

As the disease progresses, there may be widespread wasting and weakness, with bulbar dysfunction and respiratory muscle weakness.

Investigations for polymyositis and dermatomyositis include the following:

- Erythrocyte sedimentation rate (ESR)—raised.
- CK—usually raised.
- EMG—myopathic picture but may include fibrillations.

- Muscle biopsy—muscle fiber necrosis with inflammatory infiltrate.
- Autoantibodies (e.g., antinuclear antibodies, rheumatoid factor)—present in up to 25% of patients.
- Investigation for underlying carcinoma (e.g., chest x-ray).

Corticosteroids and other immunosuppressive drugs (e.g., azathioprine, cyclophosphamide) reduce the symptoms in about 75% of cases of polymyositis and dermatomyositis that are not associated with malignancy. Removal of an associated tumor may cause complete remission.

There is full recovery in about 10% of patients. The remainder have varying degrees of disability, and the disease may become inactive after a few years. When associated with connective tissue disease, the prognosis is linked to the course of this disease.

Common investigations and causes of acquired myopathies	
Investigation	**Cause of myopathy**
complete blood count and ESR	polymyositis systemic connective tissue disease carcinoma
electrolytes and renal function tests	hypokalemia (diuretics or laxatives) renal disease Cushing's syndrome
liver function tests	alcohol abuse chronic liver disease
calcium; phosphate; alkaline phosphatase	vitamin D deficiency
thyroid function tests	thyrotoxicosis hypothyroidism
cortisol studies	Cushing's disease
creatine kinase (CK)	raised in many myopathies
CXR; abdominal ultrasound; mammogram	underlying carcinoma
history of drugs or toxins	alcohol steroids clofibrate chloroquine zidovudine (AZT) lipid-lowering statins

Fig. 30.5 Common investigations and causes of acquired myopathies.

181

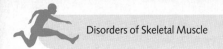

Acquired metabolic and endocrine myopathies

A wide range of diseases (especially endocrine diseases), acquired biochemical abnormalities, and drugs can result in myopathy. The weakness tends to be proximal. Most cases are reversible with treatment of the primary condition or removal of the drug.

Fig. 30.5 lists some general medical investigations that may be necessary in patients with acquired myopathy of unknown cause.

31. Vascular Diseases of the Nervous System

Cerebrovascular disease

Cerebrovascular disease is a major cause of mortality and morbidity in the developed world. Strokes of all types rank third as a cause of death, surpassed only by heart disease and cancer.

Definitions
Stroke
Stroke is a focal, nonconvulsive, neurologic deficit caused by a vascular lesion. The onset is sudden, and the symptoms last longer than 24 hours, if the patient survives.

Thromboembolic disease accounts for 85% of strokes. The most common presentation is hemiplegia caused by occlusion of the contralateral middle cerebral artery. Strokes due to intracerebral hemorrhage caused by rupture of microaneurysms (Charcot–Bouchard aneurysms), usually secondary to hypertension, are less common, but it is often difficult to distinguish them clinically from thromboembolic strokes.

Transient ischemic attack (TIA)
A TIA is a focal, nonconvulsive, neurologic deficit lasting less than 24 hours, with complete clinical recovery, caused by focal hypoperfusion within the brain. Examples of the types of deficits that can occur are listed in Fig. 31.1. The symptoms are often recurrent, and repeated episodes are often stereotypical. The onset of symptoms is usually sudden.

Almost one-third of patients who have a TIA will develop a disabling stroke within 5 years; the majority of strokes will occur within 18 months. Therefore, prompt investigation and preventive strategies are essential.

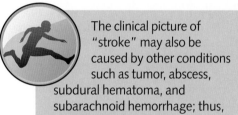

The clinical picture of "stroke" may also be caused by other conditions such as tumor, abscess, subdural hematoma, and subarachnoid hemorrhage; thus, any unusual features in the history and examination must be further investigated.

Incidence
The incidence of stroke is 600,000 per year in the U.S. The incidence is higher in African Americans than in Caucasians.

The incidence of TIA is 50–100 cases per 100,000 persons per year.

The rates increase markedly with advancing age.

Etiology of stroke
The causes of stroke are as follows (the first three are responsible for the majority of cases):
- Atherosclerosis—causes thromboembolic stroke from large extracranial arteries, most commonly the carotid arteries, or from intracranial arteries.
- Cardiac embolism—from a variety of cardiac sources, especially atrial fibrillation.
- Intracerebral hemorrhage—most often secondary to hypertension but can be caused by other factors (e.g., trauma, anticoagulant therapy, amyloid angiopathy, neoplasia, and coagulation disorders such as hemophilia or abnormalities of platelet number or function).
- Lipohyalinosis of small arteries that penetrate the brain substance—occurs in patients with

Clinical features of TIAs	
Anterior circulation (carotid arteries)	**Posterior circulation** (vertebrobasilar arteries)
amaurosis fugax	diplopia, vertigo
aphasia	dysarthria/dysphagia
contralateral hemiparesis	unilateral/bilateral or
contralateral	alternating paresis or
homonymous visual	sensory loss
field loss	binocular visual loss
any combination of the	ataxia
above	loss of consciousness (rare)
	any combination of the
	above

Fig. 31.1 Clinical features of transient ischemic attacks (TIAs).

hypertension. Occlusion of these penetrating arteries causes subcortical infarcts, less than 1.5 cm in length, which are called lacunes.

- Diseases of the vessel wall—much rarer but should always be considered in young patients who present with stroke. Causes include rheumatoid vasculitis, systemic lupus erythematosus (SLE), polyarteritis nodosa, temporal arteritis, and sarcoidosis.

> Prevention of cerebrovascular disease by identifying and controlling risk factors has a greater effect in the reduction of death and disability than any medical or surgical intervention once a stroke has occurred.

Risk factors

Risk factors include:

- Hypertension—a major factor in the development of thrombotic and hemorrhagic stroke and lacunar infarcts.
- Diabetes mellitus—increases the risk of cerebral infarction twofold and should be aggressively treated as it is a recognized risk factor for atherosclerosis.
- Cardiac disease—in addition to cardiac causes of embolic strokes (e.g., atrial fibrillation,

cardiomyopathy, arrhythmias, and valve disease), the presence of coronary artery disease is a marker for atherosclerosis elsewhere and is therefore a marker for stroke.

- Hyperlipidemia—less significant for stroke than for coronary artery disease.
- Smoking—cessation of smoking lowers the risk of ischemic stroke.
- Family history—close relatives are at slightly greater risk than nongenetically related family members of a stroke patient. Diabetes and hypertension show familial propensity, thus clouding the significance of pure hereditary factors.
- Obesity and diet—probably less significant for stroke than for coronary artery disease.
- Oral contraceptive—may increase risk of thromboembolic stroke, cerebral venous thrombosis, and subarachnoid hemorrhage in vulnerable individuals.

Vascular anatomy

It is important to know the arterial supply of the brain and the common sites of atheromatous plaques in order to appreciate the various presentations of cerebrovascular disease and their significance.

The circle of Willis (Fig. 31.2) is supplied anteriorly by the two carotid arteries and posteriorly by the basilar artery, which is formed by the union of the two vertebral arteries.

The most common sites for extracranial atheromatous plaques are:

- The origin of the internal carotid arteries.
- Within the carotid syphon.
- The origin of the vertebral arteries.

From the circle of Willis arise the anterior, middle, and posterior cerebral arteries, which supply specific portions of the cerebral hemispheres (Fig. 31.3); thus, reduction in perfusion in each territory will cause different and specific deficits.

The most commonly involved artery is the middle cerebral artery. As well as supplying the motor and sensory cortices bilaterally, which control the contralateral side of the body, the middle cerebral artery supplies the areas of the cortex pertaining to the comprehension (Wernicke's area) and expression (Broca's area) of speech (see Fig. 31.3). These areas are found in the dominant hemisphere only; thus, in the majority of right-handed individuals, speech will

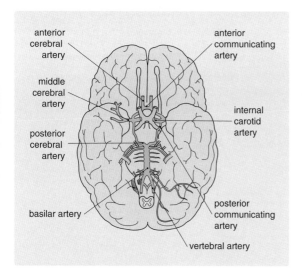

Fig. 31.2 The circle of Willis.

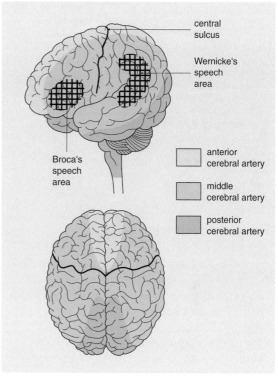

Fig. 31.3 The distribution of the three major cerebral arteries (lateral and tomographic views).

be affected only when there is occlusion of the left middle cerebral artery.

Clinical syndromes
Anterior cerebral artery occlusion
The anterior cerebral artery is a branch of the internal carotid artery and runs above the optic nerve to follow the curve of the corpus callosum. The two arteries are linked by the anterior communicating artery and thus the effect of occlusion depends on the relation with respect to the anterior communicating artery (see Fig. 31.2). Occlusion proximal to the anterior communicating artery is normally well tolerated because of adequate cross-flow, and thus few symptoms result. Occlusion distal to the anterior communicating artery causes contralateral weakness and cortical sensory loss in the lower limb (see Fig. 13.1 and Fig 14.1). Often incontinence is present and occasionally a contralateral grasp reflex.

Middle cerebral artery occlusion
The middle cerebral artery is the largest branch of the internal carotid artery and supplies the largest area of the cerebral cortex (see Fig. 31.3).

The most common form of stroke is caused by infarction of the internal capsule subsequent to thromboembolic disease within this branch of the middle cerebral artery.

Although this is a very small area, a number of extremely important structures pass through this

space, including the pyramidal tracts, sensory pathways, and the optic radiation.

> The upper part of the face is supplied bilaterally by the cerebral hemispheres; thus upper motor neuron lesions will only cause weakness of the lower part of the face. If there is marked weakness of eye closure and eyebrow lifting, a lower motor neuron or seventh cranial nerve lesion has occurred.

The signs of a middle cerebral artery occlusion are listed in Fig. 31.4. Initially, the limbs are flaccid and areflexic. After a variable period, the reflexes recover and become exaggerated, and the plantar responses become extensor, with spastic limb tone. There is variable recovery of weakness over the course of days, weeks, or months.

185

Signs of middle cerebral artery occlusion
contralateral hemiplegia (including the lower part of the face)
contralateral cortical hemisensory loss
dominant hemisphere (usually left): aphasia
nondominant hemisphere: neglect of contralateral limb dressing apraxia
contralateral homonymous hemianopia

Fig. 31.4 Signs of middle cerebral artery occlusion.

Posterior cerebral artery occlusion

The posterior cerebral arteries are the terminal branches of the basilar artery. In addition to cortical branches to the temporal lobe and occipital and visual cortices, there are perforating branches which supply the midbrain and thalamus.

The effect of occlusion depends on the site:

- Proximal occlusion: midbrain syndrome (Weber's syndrome)—third nerve palsy and contralateral hemiplegia; thalamic syndrome; chorea or hemiballismus; hemisensory disturbance.
- Cortical vessel occlusion: homonymous hemianopia with macular sparing. (The macular area is supplied by the middle cerebral artery.)
- Bilateral occlusion: Anton's syndrome (cortical blindness). The patient is blind but lacks insight into the degree of visual loss and often denies it.

Brainstem stroke

With brainstem stroke, multiple patterns of deficit can arise, depending on the exact location of the lesion with respect to the long tracts, brainstem connections, and cranial nerve nuclei. As a result of the vascular supply, unilateral lesions are more likely in the midbrain and pons, and bilateral lesions are possible in the medulla. Possible clinical features are summarized in Fig. 31.5.

Specific brainstem syndromes
Lateral medullary syndrome (posterior inferior cerebellar artery [PICA] syndrome; Wallenberg's syndrome)

Lateral medullar syndrome is the most widely recognized brainstem syndrome. Clinical features include sudden-onset vertigo (eighth cranial nerve), vomiting, ipsilateral ataxia, ipsilateral facial numbness (fifth cranial nerve), nystagmus, ipsilateral

Features of brainstem infarction	
Clinical features	**Structures involved**
upper motor neuron hemiparesis or tetraparesis	corticospinal tracts (pyramidal tracts)
hemisensory or bilateral sensory impairment	medial lemniscus or spinothalamic tracts
diplopia	3rd, 4th (midbrain) cranial nerve, and/or 6th (pons) nuclei or their connections, e.g., median longitudinal fasciculus
facial sensory loss	5th cranial nerve nucleus (midbrain, pons, medulla)
lower motor neuron facial weakness (upper and lower face)	7th nerve nucleus (pons)
nystagmus, vertigo	vestibular nuclei (pons and medulla) and connections
dysphagia, dysarthria	9th and 10th cranial nerves nuclei (medulla)
dysarthria, ataxia, vomiting, hiccoughs	cerebellum and cerebellar brainstem connections
Horner's syndrome (miosis, ptosis, enophthalmos, and disturbed sweating)	sympathetic fibers in lateral brainstem
altered consciousness	reticular formation

Fig. 31.5 Features of brainstem infarction.

Horner's syndrome, and contralateral loss of pain and temperature sensation in the limbs.

"Locked-in syndrome"

"Locked-in syndrome" is caused by a bilateral infarction in the upper brainstem. The patient is conscious but mute and paralyzed. Communication is possible through eyelid blinking.

Weber's syndrome

Weber's syndrome is caused by a lesion of the basal midbrain, resulting in an ipsilateral third nerve palsy and contralateral hemiplegia (cerebral peduncle).

Clinical evaluation of strokes
History

It is essential to take a good history from the patient, if possible, or from a relative or friend. The presence of headache may indicate hemorrhage. A slowly progressive course may indicate an alternative diagnosis such as tumor with progressing edema.

Progressive loss of consciousness may indicate raised intracranial pressure secondary to a large cerebral hemorrhage or coning caused by a cerebellar hemorrhage, and must be acted upon urgently.

Risk factors

Risk factors should be elucidated and a drug history taken, especially for use of anticoagulants.

Past medical history

A history of TIAs points toward a thromboembolic stroke. A history of connective tissue disease, neoplasia, bleeding disorders, arrhythmias, and other cardiologic diseases should be sought.

Examination

In the examination, particular care should be taken to find possible causes of embolus (atrial fibrillation, carotid bruit, valve lesion, or evidence for endocarditis) and to ascertain whether the patient is or has been hypertensive and whether there is asymmetry between the two brachial pressures (evidence for subclavian stenosis).

Initial investigations

The following routine investigations should be performed:

- Complete blood count (CBC)—polycythemia; infection.
- Erythrocyte sedimentation rate (ESR); C-reactive protein (CRP)—evidence for inflammatory disease.
- Urinalysis and blood sugar—diabetes mellitus.
- Fasting lipids.
- (Blood culture—if endocarditis is suspected.)
- (Autoantibodies and coagulation studies in young patients—evidence for connective tissue disease or prothrombotic disorder, lupus anticoagulant, anticardiolipin antibody.)
- Electrocardiography (ECG)—arrhythmia or myocardial infarction.

Special investigations
Imaging

In elderly patients, in whom strokes are most common, information gained by computed tomography (CT) scanning rarely changes the management. However, if there is any doubt about the etiology of the stroke or there is the possibility of surgical intervention (e.g., cerebellar hemorrhage), a scan should be undertaken. All young patients (i.e., less than 60 years old) with strokes and TIAs should have a CT or magnetic resonance imaging (MRI) and MR angiography (MRA).

Carotid Doppler

Carotid Doppler is an extremely effective, noninvasive means of demonstrating internal carotid artery stenosis when carotid thromboembolism is suspected or a carotid bruit heard. Carotid endarterectomy is considered if there is greater than 70% stenosis in a vessel which corresponds to contralateral symptoms.

Angiography

Because of the advent of carotid Doppler and MRA, conventional cerebral angiography is now used less in stroke patients; however, it is used for location of intracerebral aneurysms and for diagnosis of cerebral vasculitides. In patients with a recent completed stroke, angiography should not be considered until 1–2 weeks have elapsed.

Management of transient ischemic attacks

The management of TIAs is as follows:
- Confirm the diagnosis.
- Investigate possible sites of the primary lesion (e.g., carotid stenosis, cardiac embolus secondary to atrial fibrillation).
- Identify and treat risk factors (e.g., reduce hypertension).
- Aspirin—reduces platelet aggregation and should be routinely used (unless contraindications exist) to reduce the risk of further events.
- Antiplatelet agents—clopidogrel (Plavix) and ticlopidine (Ticlid) are effective alternatives to aspirin. Ticlopidine has been associated with neutropenia.
- Anticoagulation (heparin and warfarin)—not to be encouraged routinely because use of anticoagulants can precipitate hemorrhagic stroke and cause hemorrhage into an infarct; however, they are indicated in patients with a known cardiac source of embolus and atrial fibrillation, once a scan has excluded hemorrhage.

Management of a completed stroke

The management of a completed stroke is mainly supportive at present, although trials of thrombolytic agents are being carried out.

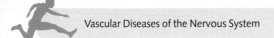

The management aims are as follows:
- Confirm diagnosis (history, examination, and investigations).
- Prevent progression of present event.
- Prevent development of complications (e.g., aspiration pneumonia, pressure sores, deep vein thrombosis).
- Rehabilitate the patient (e.g., physiotherapy, occupational therapy, and speech therapy).
- Control hypertension.
- Encourage the patient to stop smoking.
- Correct lipid abnormality.
- Good glycemic control in diabetic patients.
- Give aspirin.
- Remove or treat embolic source (e.g., anticoagulation, antibiotics for endocarditis, or endarterectomy). Note: Anticoagulation is indicated for cardiac embolus but only once hemorrhage has been excluded and not for at least 5 days after an acute event (to prevent a hemorrhagic infarct).
- Treat inflammatory or connective tissue diseases.
- Stop thrombogenic drugs (e.g., oral contraceptives).

Tissue plasminogen activator (TPA)

TPA is approved for treatment of acute ischemic stroke. The key is delivery within 3 hours of stroke onset.

Contraindications include:
- CT evidence of hemorrhage.
- Seizure at onset of stroke.
- Systolic blood pressure > 185 mmHg or diastolic pressure > 110 mmHg.
- Platelets < 100,000.
- Glucose < 50 mg/dL or > 400 mg/dL.
- Rapidly progressive symptoms.

Prognosis

One-fourth of patients die within the first month following a stroke. The mortality is greater in patients with intracerebral hemorrhage.

A worse prognosis is indicated by coma, defects in conjugate gaze, and severe hemiplegia.

There is a 10% recurrence of stroke within the first year.

There is a further 60–70% mortality rate within 3 years resulting from complications (e.g., chest infection, pulmonary embolus) and from other atherosclerotic disease (e.g., myocardial infarction).

Among the survivors, gradual improvement usually occurs, but many are left with severe residual deficits. About one-third return to independent mobility.

Intracranial hemorrhage

Intracranial hemorrhage can be subdivided by site:
- Primary intracerebral hemorrhage (considered in the section on cerebrovascular disease).
- Subarachnoid hemorrhage.
- Subdural and extradural hemorrhage.

Subarachnoid hemorrhage

Subarachnoid hemorrhage is caused by spontaneous (rather than traumatic) arterial bleeding into the subarachnoid space.

Incidence

The incidence of subarachnoid hemorrhage is 12 cases per 100,000 persons per year in North America. The incidence is highest in Japan.

Causes

Causes of subarchnoid hemorrhage comprise:
- Saccular ("berry") aneurysms—70%.
- Arteriovenous malformations (AVMs)—10%.
- Not defined—20%.

Clinical features

The clinical features of subarachnoid hemorrhage are as follows:
- Severe headache of instantaneous onset ("worst headache of my life").
- Transient or prolonged loss of consciousness or seizure may follow immediately.
- Nausea and vomiting often occur.
- Drowsiness or coma may continue for hours to days.
- Signs of meningism occur after 3–12 hours (neck stiffness on passive flexion; positive Kernig's sign [lifting the leg and extending the knee with the patient lying supine stretches the nerve roots and causes meningeal pain]).
- Focal signs from a hematoma may be present (e.g., limb weakness, aphasia).
- Papilledema may be present and may be accompanied by subhyaloid and vitreous hemorrhage.

Investigation

CT scanning is the investigation of choice and usually shows subarachnoid or intraventricular blood.

Lumbar puncture should be carried out if a CT scan is not available or if the scan is inconclusive. The diagnosis of subarachnoid hemorrhage can be made when the cerebrospinal fluid (CSF) is xanthochromic (straw-colored supernatant), which occurs due to breakdown products of hemoglobin but takes at least 6 hours.

Angiography is carried out at the earliest convenience, but delayed in patients with a poor clinical condition. Angiograms are required to localize aneurysms and arteriovenous malformations.

Immediate management

Immediate management of a subarachnoid hemorrhage includes:

- Regular neurologic observations.
- Bed rest and fluid replacement.
- Analgesia for headache—codeine or dihydrocodeine (stronger analgesics may depress conscious level and mask deterioration).
- Nimodipine (a calcium-channel blocker)—reduces vasospasm and thus mortality.
- Control of hypertension (but care should be taken to avoid hypotension, which can cause deterioration.)
- Transfer to neurosurgical intensive care unit.

Subsequent management

Once the patient is stabilized, an angiogram is carried out to localize the cause.

Berry aneurysms are the most common finding. For many patients, an endovascular approach is optimal. Emergent angiography, followed by endovascular coils, is completed to prompt occlusion. An alternative treatment is neurosurgical clipping of the aneurysm.

AVMs can be treated conservatively or with direct surgery, radiosurgery, or embolization.

Prognosis

There is a mortality rate of almost 50% before arrival at the hospital. Of patients surviving the initial bleed, 30% die within 3 months; of these, 10–20% from further bleeding within the first month. Almost half of the survivors make a good recovery.

Operative mortality ranges from 5% to 50%, depending on the patient's clinical condition and the timing of surgery.

Prognostic guides include age, quantity of subarachnoid blood on CT scan, loss of consciousness at ictus, clinical condition on admission, and presence of preexisting hypertension or arterial disease.

Subdural and epidural hemorrhage

Both subdural and extradural hemorrhages can be fatal unless treated promptly.

Subdural hematoma

Subdural hematoma results from rupture of cortical veins bridging the dura and brain and is almost invariably caused by trauma to the head.

In an acute subdural hemorrhage, there can be rapid accumulation of blood with a space-occupying effect, leading to rapid transtentorial herniation.

With a chronic subdural hematoma, the initial injury may be minor and there may be a latent interval, from days to months, between injury and symptoms. Chronic subdural hematoma is common in the elderly and in alcoholics. Symptoms can be indolent and fluctuate and include headache, drowsiness, and confusion. However, focal deficits, seizures, stupor, and coma can occur.

Epidural hemorrhage

Epidural hemorrhage is caused by a traumatic tear in the middle meningeal artery, usually associated with a temporal or parietal skull fracture.

Blood accumulates rapidly in the epidural spaces, over minutes to hours. After a lucid period, the patient may then develop focal signs, coma, and transtentorial herniation, leading to death.

Management

Diagnosis is confirmed by CT scan (Fig. 31.6).

Urgent surgical drainage is undertaken for acute subdural or extradural hematoma. Chronic subdural hematoma is often evacuated through burr holes.

Cerebrovascular involvement in vasculitis and connective tissue diseases

The vasculitides and connective tissue diseases cause inflammation and necrosis of blood vessels, and cerebral involvement can be part of a generalized systemic disease or may be isolated (Fig. 31.7).

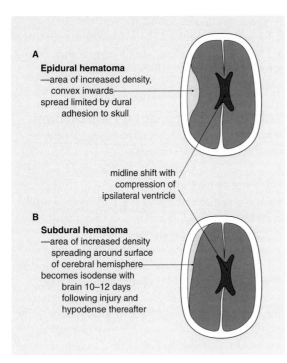

A

Epidural hematoma
—area of increased density, convex inwards—spread limited by dural adhesion to skull

midline shift with compression of ipsilateral ventricle

B

Subdural hematoma
—area of increased density spreading around surface of cerebral hemisphere—becomes isodense with brain 10–12 days following injury and hypodense thereafter

Fig. 31.6 (A) Epidural hematoma biconvex, high-density lesion abutting the inner margin of the skull. Midline ventricular shift and sulcal effacement can occur in both subdural and extradural hematomas if they are sufficiently large. (B) Subdural hematoma—crescent-shaped, high-density lesion lying adjacent to the inner margin of skull. As the hematoma ages, it can become isodense with the brain substance.

All of these conditions can cause stroke (infarction or hemorrhage) and should be considered in any young patient with stroke or any patient with unusual or systemic features.

Many of the conditions can present with other signs of neurologic involvement of either the central or peripheral nervous system.

Investigations

Investigations should include ESR, CRP, autoantibodies, imaging (CT/MRI), angiography (direct or MRI), CSF, and, if appropriate, biopsy of the skin, blood vessel, or meninges.

Treatment

Treatment is with steroids and immunosuppressive drugs, depending on the disease.

Connective tissue diseases and vasculitides that can present with stroke	
Connective tissue diseases	**Vasculitides**
• systemic lupus erythematosus (SLE) • rheumatoid arthritis • Sjögren's syndrome	• systemic necrotizing vasculitis—polyarteritis nodosa • Wegener's granulomatosis • giant-cell arteritis—temporal arteritis; Takayasu's arteritis • Behçet's disease • granulomatous angiitis

Fig. 31.7 Connective tissue diseases and vasculitides that can present with stroke.

Cerebral venous thrombosis

Blood from the brain is drained by cerebral veins, which empty into dural sinuses, which subsequently drain into the internal jugular veins.

Venous sinus thrombosis is associated with:
- Infection—local drainage (middle ear, paranasal sinuses, face) and generalized.
- Head injury.
- Dehydration,
- Pregnancy, puerperium, oral contraception.
- Hematologic diseases (e.g., polycythemia).
- Malignant meningitis.
- Inflammatory disorders (e.g., Behçet's disease, sarcoidosis, SLE).

The superior sagittal sinus is most commonly involved, followed by the lateral sinus and cavernous sinus, although all are rare.

Clinical features

The clinical features of thrombosis in the major sinuses and cerebral veins are variable. The most common presentations are headache, motor and sensory deficit, seizures, mental changes, and papilledema.

Cavernous sinus thrombosis

Cavernous sinus thrombosis warrants special mention because of its distinctive clinical picture. The cavernous sinus (Fig. 31.8) drains venous blood from the eye, and many important structures run by or through it, including the carotid artery and the

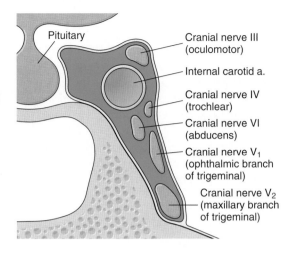

Fig. 31.8 Coronal section of cavernous sinus.

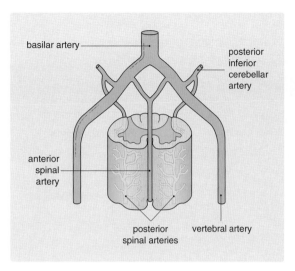

Fig. 31.9 Vascular supply of the spinal cord.

third, fourth, fifth (ophthalmic division), and sixth cranial nerves. Classic, acute cases of cavernous sinus thrombosis are associated with proptosis, chemosis, and painful ophthalmoplegia.

Diagnosis
MRI and MRA are now the key procedures for diagnosis of cerebral venous thrombosis.

Treatment
Treatment regimens for cerebral venous thrombosis remain controversial and vary in different centers. They are based on symptomatic treatment (e.g., anticonvulsants, antibiotics, and methods to reduce intracranial pressure) and on anticoagulation with heparin.

Spinal cord vascular disease

The blood supply to the spinal cord is complex. The main vessels are the paired posterior spinal arteries, which run down the posterior surface of the cord, and the single anterior spinal artery, which runs down the median fissure anteriorly (Fig. 31.9).

During development, five to eight radicular arteries become predominant and provide most of the flow to the spinal cord through the anterior spinal artery. The largest is the artery of Adamkiewicz, which enters at the T9–T11 level and supplies the major portion of blood to the lower thoracic cord and lumbar enlargement.

The midthoracic region is most vulnerable because the supply to the anterior spinal artery often consists of only one significant radicular artery and because there is a poor anastomotic network at this level.

The posterior spinal arteries have a rich collateral supply and therefore the posterior part of the cord is relatively protected from the effects of vascular disease.

Fig 31.10 shows the vascular supply of the cord in cross section and therefore indicates the supply of the major pathways.

Anterior spinal artery syndrome
If the anterior spinal artery becomes occluded, the supply to the anterior two thirds of the cord is disrupted causing anterior spinal artery syndrome, resulting in disruption of the corticospinal and spinothalamic tracts bilaterally (see Fig. 31.10).

Because the posterior spinal arteries, which supply the posterior columns, have a rich collateral supply, they are relatively protected from vascular disease. There is virtually no anastomotic connection between the anterior and posterior territories.

Causes
Causes of anterior spinal artery syndrome include:
- Small-vessel disease (e.g., diabetes, polyarteritis, SLE).
- Arterial compression or occlusion (e.g., disc fragments, epidural mass, dissecting aortic aneurysm, aortic surgery).

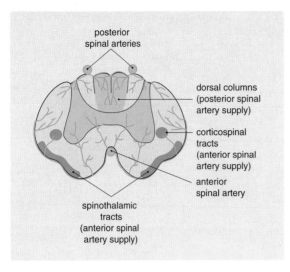

Fig. 31.10 Cross-sectional view of the vascular supply of the spinal cord.

- Embolism (e.g., aortic angiography, decompression sickness).
- Hypotension—the arterial watershed at the midthoracic region is especially susceptible to hypoperfusion.

Clinical features

The clinical features of anterior spinal artery syndrome are dependent on the level of the lesion and include:
- Segmental pain at onset—usually in the back and around the trunk.
- Sphincter disturbance—usually urinary retention, but incontinence of bladder and bowel can occur.
- Flaccid paraparesis, which progresses to spasticity over days (corticospinal tracts). Tetraparesis is less common, as the thoracic cord is most vulnerable.
- Areflexia below the level of the lesion, which progresses to hyperreflexia and extensor plantar responses over days.
- Loss of pain and temperature sensation up to the dermatome level at which the lesion occurred (spinothalamic tracts).
- Vibration and joint-position sense are intact because the dorsal columns are supplied by the posterior spinal artery.

Management

Treatment is symptomatic. The prognosis for recovery is variable but usually poor.

32. Intracranial Tumors

Intracranial tumors can be defined as benign or malignant expanding lesions within the cranial cavity. They can be:

- Primary (e.g., gliomas, meningiomas, neurofibromas).
- Secondary—metastatic carcinoma (e.g., lung, breast) or lymphoma.

Primary intracranial tumors account for approximately 10% of all neoplasms. They can be derived from neuroepithelial cells (gliomas), the meninges, nerve sheath cells, the anterior pituitary, or blood vessels.

Types of intracranial tumor

The relative frequencies of the most common intracranial tumors are shown in Fig. 32.1.

Gliomas

Gliomas are malignant, intrinsic tumors originating in neuroglia, usually within the cerebral hemispheres. They virtually never metastasize outside the central nervous system (CNS) and spread only by direct extension.

There are many different types. The most common are presented below.

Astrocytoma

Astrocytomas arise from astrocytes and are the most common primary brain tumor. They can be separated histologically into four grades dependent on the degree of malignancy (grade I—pilocytic; slow growing over years; grade IV—glioblastoma multiforme; death within months).

Oligodendroglioma

Oligodendrogliomas arise from oligodendrocytes and form slow-growing, sharply defined tumors that may become calcified. Variants include an anaplastic form and a mixed astrocytoma/oligodendroglioma.

Ependymoma

Derived from ependymal cells and choroid plexus, ependymomas can arise anywhere throughout the ventricular system or spinal canal. They spread through cerebrospinal pathways and infiltrate surrounding tissue.

Meningiomas

Meningiomas are benign tumors that arise from the arachnoid membrane and may grow to a large size, usually over many years. They tend to compress adjacent brain structures rather than infiltrate. Calcification is common. They are rare below the tentorium.

Pituitary tumors

Pituitary tumors may cause endocrine dysfunction that is not always apparent to the patient. They may also present with visual symptoms due to chiasmal compression, resulting classically in a bitemporal hemianopia. If untreated, the visual failure may progress and become irreversible.

The most common types of pituitary tumor include:

- Prolactinomas—chromophobe adenomas.
- Nonfunctioning chromophobe adenomas.
- Acidophil adenomas—acromegaly.
- Basophil adenomas or hyperplasia—Cushing's disease or Nelson's syndrome.

Neurofibromas and schwannomas

Neurofibromas and schwannomas arise from Schwann cells. The principal intracranial site is in the cerebellopontine angle, where they arise from the eighth cranial nerve sheath (Fig. 32.2). This is a common finding in neurofibromatosis type 2 but is usually sporadic. Clinical features of an acoustic schwannoma include ipsilateral sensory deafness, ipsilateral fifth and seventh nerve palsies and ipsilateral cerebellar signs. Ultimately, contralateral pyramidal signs may develop.

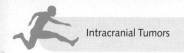

Relative frequencies of the commonest intracranial tumors	
Tumor	Relative frequency (%)
malignant—gliomas (especially astrocytomas and oligodendrogliomas)	40
metastases	25
meningiomas	15
pituitary adenomas	10
neurofibromas/schwannomas	5
others	15

Fig. 32.1 The relative frequencies of the most common intracranial tumors.

Hemangioblastomas

Hemangioblastomas are derived from blood vessels and occur within the cerebellar parenchyma or spinal cord. They are found in Von Hippel–Lindau disease in association with similar tumors in the retina and cystic lesions in the pancreas.

Clinical features of intracranial tumors

Mass lesions within the cranium may present with one or more of the following features:

- Effects of raised intracranial pressure—headache, vomiting, papilledema.
- Focal neurologic signs occurring singly or in various combinations, caused by the direct effects of the tumor (compression, infiltration, or edema).
- Diffuse cerebral symptoms—seizures, cognitive impairment.

Intracranial tumors, primary and secondary, are the most common cause of these symptoms, but any space-occupying lesion can present similarly (e.g., cerebral abscess, tuberculoma, subdural or intracerebral hematoma).

Raised intracranial pressure

Raised intracranial pressure produces the classic triad of headache, vomiting, and papilledema. However, these features, especially papilledema, are relatively infrequent presentations early on, as the symptoms usually imply obstruction to the cerebrospinal

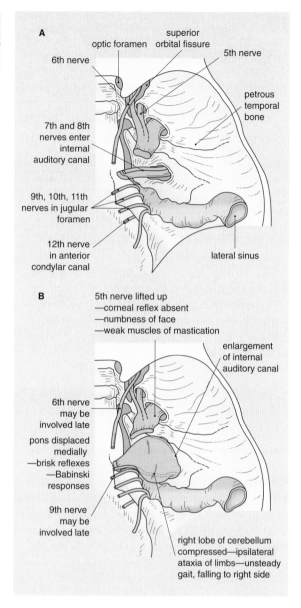

Fig. 32.2 Acoustic neuroma.

pathways. The full picture is more common early in posterior fossa tumors.

The raised pressure caused by the expanding mass and resultant edema causes symptoms and signs distant to the tumor, including:

- Herniation.
- False localizing signs.

Herniation

There may be compression of the medulla by herniation of the cerebellar tonsils through the

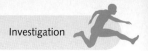

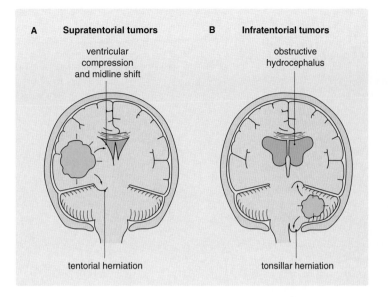

Fig. 32.3 Herniation of (A) the temporal lobe (supratentorial tumors) and (B) the cerebellar tonsils (infratentorial tumors; coning).

foramen magnum, which leads to impairment of consciousness, respiratory depression, bradycardia, decerebrate posturing, and death (Fig. 32.3).

Similarly, the uncus of the temporal lobe may herniate through the tentorial opening (see Fig. 32.3). A pupil-involved third nerve palsy may result in addition to other signs. The nerve is compressed against the petroclinoid ligament and causes displacement of the posterior communicating artery.

False localizing signs

These are "false" in that they are distant to the site of the mass and caused by the raised pressure. They include:

- Sixth nerve palsy—caused by compression of the nerve during its long intracranial course. It is often unilateral initially, then bilateral.
- Third nerve palsy—caudal herniation of the uncus of the temporal lobe causes pupillary dilatation and then later ophthalmoplegia.
- Hemiparesis on the same side as the tumor—caused by compression of the brainstem on the free edge of the tentorium (Kernohan's notch).

False localizing signs are very important because they indicate an increase in pressure with brain shift and require urgent response, which may be surgical.

Focal neurologic signs

Focal neurologic signs may be caused by direct effects of the tumor (compression, infiltration, or edema) or be false localizing signs (as discussed above). The direct effects will depend on the site of the tumor (Fig. 32.4).

Seizures

Partial seizures, whether simple or complex, are characteristic of many hemispheric lesions. They may then secondarily generalize to a tonic-clonic seizure. They are often difficult to control.

Investigation

If an intracranial tumor is suspected, imaging is essential. However, as many intracranial tumors are metastatic, generalized, routine investigations are also necessary (e.g., chest x-ray).

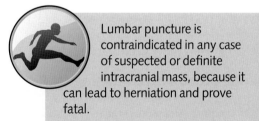

Lumbar puncture is contraindicated in any case of suspected or definite intracranial mass, because it can lead to herniation and prove fatal.

Computed tomography (CT)

CT scans should be carried out with contrast, as enhancement of a lesion (which may not be visible precontrast) adds to the discriminating ability. However, CT scans only show the presence and site

195

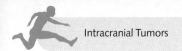

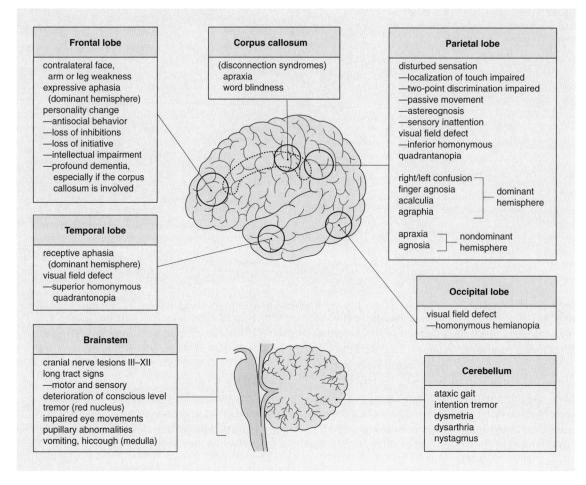

Frontal lobe

contralateral face,
arm or leg weakness
expressive aphasia
(dominant hemisphere)
personality change
—antisocial behavior
—loss of inhibitions
—loss of initiative
—intellectual impairment
—profound dementia,
especially if the corpus
callosum is involved

Corpus callosum

(disconnection syndromes)
apraxia
word blindness

Parietal lobe

disturbed sensation
—localization of touch impaired
—two-point discrimination impaired
—passive movement
—astereognosis
—sensory inattention
visual field defect
—inferior homonymous
quadrantanopia

right/left confusion ⎤
finger agnosia   ⎥ dominant
acalculia   ⎥ hemisphere
agraphia   ⎦

apraxia ⎤ nondominant
agnosia ⎦ hemisphere

Temporal lobe

receptive aphasia
(dominant hemisphere)
visual field defect
—superior homonymous
quadrantonopia

Occipital lobe

visual field defect
—homonymous hemianopia

Brainstem

cranial nerve lesions III–XII
long tract signs
—motor and sensory
deterioration of conscious level
tremor (red nucleus)
impaired eye movements
pupillary abnormalities
vomiting, hiccough (medulla)

Cerebellum

ataxic gait
intention tremor
dysmetria
dysarthria
nystagmus

Fig. 32.4 Focal neurologic signs according to the site of the tumor.

of a mass, and whether there is edema, shift, or hydrocephalus, but do not indicate its nature. Different intracranial masses—i.e., tumors (benign and malignant), cerebral abscesses, and tuberculomas—all have characteristic, but not entirely diagnostic, appearances (Fig. 32.5).

Magnetic resonance imaging (MRI)
MRI usually provides more anatomical information than CT scanning and is always the investigation of choice for suspected posterior fossa mass lesions. Small metastases and meningeal lesions may also be missed by CT scans.

Electroencephalography (EEG)
EEG is rarely indicated or helpful in the investigation of tumors. There may be abnormal electrical activity

in the region of the mass, but the EEG may be normal.

Skull x-ray
Skull x-ray is rarely indicated except to define bony landmarks or pathology in selected cases prior to surgery.

Specialized neuroradiology
Angiograms may be required to define the site and blood supply of a mass and ensure that it is not vascular in nature.

Stereotactic brain biopsy
A frame is positioned on the head with identifiable external reference (fiducial) markers. With the use of CT or MRI, insertion of a cannula at any point

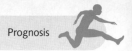

Fig. 32.5 CT scan features of various intracranial tumors.

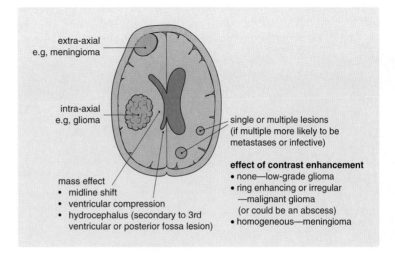

selected on the image can be performed, to allow biopsy. The subsequent histological findings will help determine further management.

Treatment

Cerebral edema
The edema surrounding the tumor can be reduced with the use of corticosteroids (dexamethasone) or mannitol.

Seizures
Seizures are treated with antiepileptic drugs but are often difficult to control.

Surgery
Benign tumors can often be entirely removed. This is usually difficult with malignant tumors, which are usually debulked.

Radiotherapy
Radiotherapy is usually recommended for gliomas and radiosensitive metastases.

Chemotherapy
Chemotherapy is often of little therapeutic value in primary brain tumors. Wafers impregnated with chemotherapy can be placed within the brain and are currently under investigation.

Prognosis

The prognosis for malignant brain tumors is poor. There is an overall 1-year survival of less than 50%. Benign tumors, especially meningiomas and neurofibromas, are often removed entirely and therefore cured.

33. Infections of the Nervous System

This chapter will consider only the most common and important infections of the nervous system.

General conditions will be considered first, followed by diseases caused by individual organisms.

General conditions

Meningitis

Definition

Meningitis is an inflammation of the meninges (the pia and arachnoid and the cerebrospinal fluid that they enclose).

The term typically refers to inflammation caused by an infective agent; however, it can also be applied to inflammation of the meninges caused by malignant cells, drugs, contrast media, and blood following subarachnoid hemorrhage. All of these causes can have a similar presentation to infective causes.

Infective agents can reach the meninges from direct spread (e.g., from sinuses or the nasopharynx), through fractures of the skull, or, more commonly, from the bloodstream.

Causative agents

Meningitis can be caused by a variety of organisms, including bacteria, viruses, and fungi.

Bacteria

Among Gram-staining bacteria, the most likely causative organisms vary with age and predisposing factors.

In the neonate, they include:
- Gram-negative bacilli (e.g., *Escherichia coli*, *Klebsiella*).
- *Hemophilus influenzae*.

In children, they include:
- *Hemophilus influenzae*.
- *Streptococcus pneumoniae* (pneumococcus).
- *Neisseria meningitidis* (meningococcus).

In adults, they include:
- *Neisseria meningitidis*.
- *Streptococcus pneumoniae*.

In immunodeficiency, trauma, or neurosurgery (e.g., ventricular shunts), they include:
- *Staphylococcus aureus*.
- *Listeria monocytogenes*.
- *Proteus* species.
- Group A streptococci.

Acid-fast bacilli that can cause meningitis include *Mycobacterium tuberculosis*. Tuberculous meningitis is generally considered separately from the other bacterial meningitides as the presentation is somewhat different.

Spirochaetes causing meningitis include:
- *Treponema pallidum* (syphilis).
- *Borrelia burgdorferi* (Lyme disease).

Viruses

Viruses that can cause meningitis include:
- Enteroviruses—echovirus, coxsackievirus, and poliovirus.
- Mumps.
- Herpes simplex type II (rarely type I) and Ebstein–Barr virus (EBV).
- HIV—due to the primary infection.
- West Nile virus.

Fungi

Fungi that cause meningitis include:
- *Cryptococcus neoformans*—a common opportunistic organism in HIV-positive patients.
- *Histoplasma capsulatum*.

Clinical features

The classic clinical triad of "meningism" is:
- Headache.
- Photophobia.
- Neck stiffness.

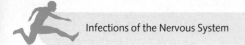

There is often a fever, with or without rigors, although with "aseptic" meningitis (i.e., not bacterial), this may be variable.

There may be a prodromal infection with myalgia and lethargy, or a likely source of infection may be evident (e.g., otitis media, pneumonia).

Bacterial meningitis

Bacterial meningitis is characterized by a sudden onset, with high fevers and rigors accompanying the classic triad. A petechial rash, which may not be very obvious, indicates meningococcal meningitis. The patient may present with septicemic shock.

Viral meningitis

Viral meningitis is acute or subacute. It is usually self-limiting and lasts 4–10 days. Headaches may last for some weeks, but serious sequelae are rare.

Tuberculous meningitis (TBM)

Tuberculosis (TB) typically causes chronic meningitis, but it may present more acutely. TBM may occur years after the primary infection. Meningitic signs may take many weeks to develop, having been preceded by nonspecific symptoms such as a vague headache, malaise, anorexia, and vomiting.

Fungal meningitis

Cryptococcal meningitis is the most common fungal meningitis in America and is especially associated with immunocompromised patients. The presentation is similar to TBM.

West Nile virus meningitis

Symptoms include hadache, fever, neck siffness, seizures, muscle weakness, and paralysis.

> Bacterial meningitis is a medical emergency with a high mortality rate. Meningococcal meningitis, in particular, can progress extremely rapidly. If there is a high index of suspicion of bacterial meningitis, and especially if a petechial rash develops (meningococcal meningitis), treatment should be started immediately, prior to confirmation of the diagnosis before lumbar puncture.

Diagnosis

Diagnosis is made by lumbar puncture. This should be carried out immediately to prevent delay in treatment. However, if there are any signs of raised intracranial pressure, a CT scan should be ordered first, because lumbar puncture could prove fatal in this situation.

Typical cerebrospinal fluid (CSF) findings are listed in Fig. 33.1. Other investigations include the following.

CSF pressure

This is characteristically elevated (>180 mm H_2O).

Staining of CSF

- Gram stain—to diagnose bacterial meningitis: Gram-positive diplococci—pneumococcus; Gram-negative intracellular diplococci—meningococcus.
- Ziehl–Nielsen stain—demonstrates acid-fast bacilli: tuberculous (acid-fast bacilli visualized in only 20% of cases of TBM).
- Indian-ink stain—stains for fungi.

Blood cultures and CSF culture

Including culture in Lowenstein–Jensen medium for TB (results take 6 weeks for TB).

Blood glucose

This is compared with CSF glucose.

Blood and CSF serology

These are carried out for likely viral causes.

Chest and skull x-rays

These are carried out (when possible) if there is a likelihood that infection has spread from the chest or via a fracture.

Complications

Consciousness is not severely impaired in uncomplicated meningitis, although a high fever may cause delirium. Marked changes in conscious level, focal neurologic signs, seizures, and papilledema indicate that complications are developing or that an alternative diagnosis should be considered (e.g., cerebral abscess or encephalitis). Complications include:

- Hydrocephalus (obstruction of CSF outflow, leading to raised intracranial pressure).
- Cerebral edema.
- Venous sinus thrombosis.
- Subdural empyema.
- Cerebral abscess.

Fig. 33.1 CSF findings in meningitis.

CSF findings in meningitis				
	Normal	**Bacterial**	**Viral**	**Tuberculous**
Appearance	clear	turbid/pus	clear/turbid	turbid/viscous
Neutrophils	nil	200–10000/mm^3	nil/few	0–200/mm^3
Lymphocytes	<5/mm^3	<50/mm^3	10–100/mm^3	100–300/mm^3
Protein	0.2–0.4g/L	0.5–2.0g/L	0.4–0.8g/L	0.5–3.0g/L
Glucose	2/3 blood glucose	<1/3 blood glucose	>1/2 blood glucose	<1/3 blood glucose

Treatment

Bacterial meningitis is a medical emergency. Each hour of delay increases the likelihood of a fatal outcome or permanent neurologic deficit.

It is usually possible to distinguish between bacterial meningitis and meningitis caused by other organisms in the clinical setting and with initial visualization of the CSF.

If there is any suspicion that a patient may have bacterial meningitis, treatment with intravenous broad-spectrum antibiotics should be started immediately—e.g., third-generation cephalosporin and vancomycin.

Tuberculous meningitis is treated for at least 9 months with a combination of isoniazid, rifampicin, and pyrazinamide, with the peripheral nerve side effects of isoniazid protected by pyridoxine. Other possible agents include ethambutol, streptomycin, and ciprofloxacin.

Viral meningitis is usually benign and self-limiting. The treatment is symptomatic.

Prophylaxis

Contacts of patients with bacterial meningitis—including family, school, and work contacts—should be considered for prophylactic treatment with oral rifampicin.

Encephalitis
Definition

Encephalitis is inflammation of the brain parenchyma, usually caused by viruses but occasionally due to bacteria or other organisms (e.g., *Mycoplasma*, *Rickettsia*, and *Histoplasma*).

The temporal course of encephalitis can differ depending on the virus. Three main forms of viral encephalitis exist:

- Direct—when the infective organism directly causes the encephalitis at the time of infection (acute viral meningoencephalitis or encephalitis).
- Delayed or latent—causing a "slow" viral encephalitis.
- Immune-mediated—causing an allergic or postinfectious encephalomyelitis, which can also follow after vaccination.

Causative organisms

The causative organisms are often not identified, and the viral etiology is presumed.

The most common organisms identified cases of adult encephalitis in the U.S. are:

- Herpes simplex—causes the most severe viral encephalitis.
- Arbovirus.
- West Nile virus.
- Eastern equine encephalitis.
- Western equine encephalitis.
- La Crosse encephalitis.
- St. Louis encephalitis.

In the Far East, the most common cause is Japanese B arbovirus, which causes epidemic encephalitis with a high mortality rate.

Clinical features

Many of the causative organisms cause a mild self-limiting illness with headache and drowsiness, but some cases present with a severe illness with depressed conscious level, focal signs, and seizures. Herpes simplex type I accounts for most of the severe cases.

Clinical features can be categorized as follows:

- Nonspecific features: headache, pyrexia, myalgia, malaise, etc.

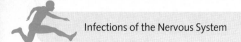

- Meningism (from meningeal involvement): headache, photophobia, neck stiffness, and lymphocytic pleocytosis in the CSF.
- Parenchymal involvement: depends whether the inflammation is diffuse or focal (e.g., confusion, aphasia, hemiparesis, seizures, ataxia, cranial nerve palsies, autonomic dysfunction).
- Virus-specific features (e.g., parotid swelling in mumps, paralysis in West Nile virus encephalitis).

Diagnosis

Definitive diagnosis is often difficult in viral encephalitis. Investigations include:

- CT scanning—often shows cerebral edema, which is nonspecific.
- MRI—can be useful to corroborate a diagnosis of herpes simplex because the virus has a predilection for the temporal lobes and the abnormality can be thus identified.
- EEG—may show nonspecific slow-wave changes and/or periodic complexes; however, if these findings are restricted to temporofrontal regions, a diagnosis of herpes simplex is suggested.
- Viral serology of blood and CSF.
- Brain biopsy—seldom performed but can provide more definitive information in difficult cases.

Treatment

Any case of suspected herpes simplex encephalitis should be treated immediately with intravenous acyclovir.

Otherwise treatment of encephalitis is supportive and symptomatic, including:

- Supportive treatment for comatose patients.
- Antiepileptic drugs for seizures.
- Control of cerebral edema.
- Use of corticosteroids for the first week of illness is controversial.

Prognosis

The prognosis is highly variable and depends on the causative organism.

In the U.S., herpes simplex carries the highest mortality rate. There is 80% mortality for untreated herpes simplex encephalitis, and the rate only falls to 30% with treatment; in contrast, the mortality for mumps encephalitis is 2%, even through there is no specific treatment.

The likelihood of neurologic sequelae is also variable and depends on the severity of the

encephalitis. Amnesia is a prominent sequel to herpes simplex encephalitis.

Cerebral abscess
Definition

A cerebral abscess is a focal area of infection within the cerebrum or cerebellum.

The abscess passes through several stages, over about 2 weeks, from localized suppurative cerebritis to complete encapsulation. There may be a solitary abscess or multiple abscesses.

The brain is relatively resistant to abscess formation, but abscesses can occur under conditions that cause necrosis of tissue with simultaneous infection by the appropriate organism.

The infection can reach the brain by local spread or via the bloodstream. Disease states that predispose to cerebral abscess formation include:

- Chronic lung infections (e.g., bronchiectasis), chronic sinusitis, otitis, or mastoiditis.
- Congenital heart disease.
- Bacterial endocarditis.
- Infections in immunocompromised patients.

Causative organisms

Bacteria are the usual causative organisms; however, in immunocompromised patients, other organisms (e.g., fungi and protozoa) are more common.

Anaerobic and microaerophylic organisms are the main pathogens:

- *Streptococcus* species, especially viridans streptococci.
- *Bacteroides* species.
- Enterobacteria (e.g., *E. coli* and *Proteus* species).
- *Staphylococcus aureus*.

In the immunocompromised patient, the following species are important:

- *Toxoplasma*.
- *Aspergillus*.
- *Candida*.
- *Listeria*.
- *Strongyloides*.

Clinical features

The history in patients with cerebral abscess is usually short (less than a month) and progressive.

Brain abscesses present as space-occupying lesions and thus with features of raised intracranial pressure:

- Headache.
- Vomiting.

- Deterioration in conscious level.
- Papilledema.

There may also be focal features associated with the space occupation:
- Seizures (occur in 30% of cases).
- Hemiparesis.
- Aphasia.
- Visual field defects.
- Ataxia.

There may also be symptoms of systemic infection (e.g., pyrexia, malaise) or of focal infection (e.g., cough, earache), but these may not be present, particularly in the immunocompromised patient.

Diagnosis

CT scanning or, if available, MRI is the investigation of choice. Lumbar puncture is contraindicated in the presence of a mass lesion because of the risk of herniation. Other investigations include x-rays of the chest, sinuses, etc., which may reveal the primary source of the infection, and blood cultures.

The classic appearance seen on a CT scan with contrast includes (Fig. 33.2):
- "Ring enhancement" of the lesion, which is usually spherical.

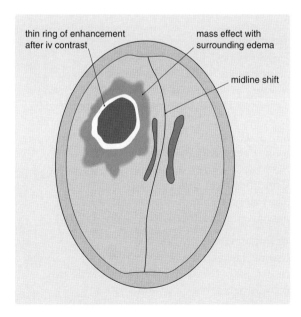

thin ring of enhancement after iv contrast

mass effect with surrounding edema

midline shift

Fig. 33.2 CT appearance of a cerebral abscess (similar appearances may be produced by an intracranial tumor).

- Central area of low density.
- Surrounding area of edema.

In addition, there may be ventricular compression and midline shift due to a mass effect.

Treatment

Treatment consists of four parts:
- Treatment of the brain abscess with appropriate antibiotics or organism-specific drugs. Often a combination is used to target all likely organisms until the organism has been isolated. For example, a third-generation cephalosporin, chloramphenicol, and metronidazole may be used for nonimmunocompromised patients, and pyrimethamine, amphotericin, and ampicillin for immunocompromised patients.
- Surgical drainage or excision of the brain abscess in association with medical treatment.
- Treatment of raised intracranial pressure and seizures.
- Treatment of the source of infection (e.g., drainage of chronic sinus infection).

Prognosis

The mortality rate since the advent of CT scanning and better bacteriologic techniques for anaerobic organisms has fallen to 5–15% (it was 30–50% prior to CT).

Poor prognostic indicators are:
- Reduced preoperative level of consciousness.
- Brain herniation.
- Rupture of the abscess into the ventricles or subarachnoid space.
- Immunocompromised patient.
- Poor general medical condition (e.g., severe pulmonary disease).

Of survivors, 25–50% have neurologic sequelae, 30–50% have persistent seizures, 15–30% have hemiparesis, and 10–20% have disorders of speech and language.

Specific organisms and the neurologic diseases that they cause

Tuberculosis

TB is an infection, which, in humans, is caused most commonly by *Mycobacterium tuberculosis*. It can

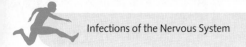
also be caused by *M. bovis*, and now, with immunosuppression secondary to HIV infection, there is an increasing incidence of cases due to *M. avium-intracellulare*.

Diagnosis
The diagnosis of neurological TB involves chest x-ray (for evidence of pulmonary TB), tuberculin testing, CSF (so long as no space-occupying lesion exists), CT scanning and MRI, and biopsy.

Treatment
Antituberculous therapy for neurologic TB should be continued for at least 12–18 months and involves a combination of isoniazid, rifampicin, pyrazinamide, and ethambutol, with pyridoxine to cover the peripheral nerve side effects of isoniazid.

Conditions caused
TB involves the nervous system in less than 1% of patients, causing the following conditions:
- Tuberculous meningitis (see p. 200).
- Tuberculoma.
- Pott's disease.
- Spinal arachnoiditis.

Tuberculoma
Tuberculoma presents as a cerebral abscess and may produce a space-occupying effect. Most cases resolve with antituberculous therapy.

Pott's disease
Tuberculous osteomyelitis of the vertebral bodies can cause chronic epidural infection. The lower thoracic region is usually involved, with pain over the affected area (which is only relieved by rest) and features of cord compression (20% of cases). Occasionally, there may be vertebral collapse or spread of infection into the pleura, peritoneum, or psoas muscle.

A needle biopsy is usually sufficient to establish the diagnosis, but occasionally exploratory surgery is required.

Treatment comprises long-term antituberculous therapy and, if signs of cord compression develop, surgical decompression.

Spinal arachnoiditis
Spinal arachnoiditis may result from downward spread of intracranial infection or from direct spread from epidural infection.

The presentation is of spreading myelitis with root involvement:

- Weakness—pyramidal and radicular.
- Root pain.
- Sensory loss.
- Sphincter disturbance.

Diagnosis is made with x-rays, myelography, and lumbar puncture.

Treatment is with antituberculous therapy and, if required, surgical decompression.

Syphilis
Syphilis is caused by the motile spirochete *Treponema pallidum* and transmission is almost invariably through sexual contact.

The natural history of untreated infection is divided into three stages. Neurologic involvement occurs in the third stage, which is typically many years after the initial infection. Neurosyphilis accounts for less than 10% of all untreated cases. Also, penicillins are widely used for the treatment of other infections, and thus many unsuspected cases of syphilis are treated without progressing to stages two and three.

Diagnosis
The serologic tests Veneral Disease Reference Laboratory (VDRL), *T. pallidum* hemagglutination assay (TPHA), and fluorescent treponema antibodies absorbed (FTA-Abs), when used in combination, provide specific results. For practical purposes, negative serology excludes the diagnosis.

Treatment
Parenteral penicillin is given for all forms of neurosyphilis for 2–3 weeks. Established neurologic disease can be arrested but may not be reversed.

Jarisch–Herxheimer reactions (severe allergic reactions due to rapid release of spirochete antigen into blood) may occur; thus, high-dose steroid cover is often given with the penicillin.

Conditions caused
The main syphilitic syndromes that affect the nervous system are described below.

Asymptomatic neurosyphilis
During the long interval between the secondary and tertiary stages of the disease, neurosyphilis may actively persist but be asymptomatic.

CSF examination reveals positive syphilis serology, lymphocytosis (100–1,000/mm^3), elevated protein (0.5–2.0g/L), and reduced glucose.

Treatment with penicillin will prevent further progression.

Meningitis

Approximately 25% of untreated patients will develop an acute symptomatic meningitis within 2 years of infection. This may present in three ways:

- Acute basal meningitis—with hydrocephalus, cranial nerve palsies, and papilledema.
- Focal meningitis—when a gumma presents as an expanding intracranial mass, favoring the meninges rather than parenchyma, and presenting with seizures, raised intracranial pressure, and focal signs.
- Meningovascular meningitis (5–10 years after primary infection)—causing an obliterative endarteritis and periarteritis and presenting as a "stroke," most often in a young person.

Treatment with penicillin will prevent progression.

Tabes dorsalis

Tabes dorsalis is a late presentation of syphilis (15–20 years after primary infection), causing a meningoradiculitis with degeneration of the dorsal columns and pupillary involvement.

The classic features include:

- Lightening pains—irregular, severe, sharp stabbing pains, usually in the lower limb, chest, or abdomen, caused by dorsal root involvement.
- Visceral crises—abdominal pain and diarrhea.
- Argyll Robertson pupils—small, irregularly shaped pupils that do not react to light but do accommodate.
- Ptosis—with compensatory overactivity of the frontalis muscle.
- Optic atrophy.
- Impaired vibration and joint-position sense, and reduced deep pain.
- Patchy loss of pinprick and temperature sensation (deafferentation).
- Trophic skin lesions and Charcot joints (painless joint damage).
- Sensory ataxia—positive Romberg's test and stamping gait.
- Hypotonia and reduced reflexes.
- Extensor plantar responses despite absent ankle jerks—caused by the combination of peripheral neuropathy and upper motor involvement.

General paralysis of the insane

General paralysis of the insane develops 10–25 years after primary infection and, as its historical name indicates, involves psychiatric abnormality and weakness. There are two phases:

- Preparalytic—with progressive dementia.
- Paralytic—with involvement of the corticospinal tracts and extrapyramidal system.

Clinical features include:

- Dementia—usually similar to that associated with Alzheimer's disease but occasionally involves manic behaviour or delusions of grandeur.
- Seizures and incontinence.
- Pupil abnormalities—pupils are large, unequal, and unreactive in 75% of cases, whereas the remainder have Argyll Robertson pupils.
- Tremor of tongue ("trombone" tongue).
- Dysarthria.
- Hypertonia with brisk reflexes and extensor plantar responses.

Human immunodeficiency virus

Infection with the retrovirus HIV can cause neurologic involvement either directly or via opportunistic infections. Neurologic involvement develops in 80% of patients.

Both the central and peripheral nervous system can be affected.

Central nervous system (CNS) involvement
Primary HIV infection

The direct effects of the virus can cause:

- HIV encephalopathy (AIDS dementia)—subacute or chronic onset.
- HIV myelopathy—a reversible form can occur during seroconversion, but a later form (when not caused by an opportunistic organism) is irreversible.
- Acute atypical meningitis—self-limiting and occurs at seroconversion, with cranial neuropathies and pyramidal signs.

Opportunistic infection

A wide variety of organisms may be responsible. The most common conditions include:

- CNS toxoplasmosis—the most commonly encountered neurologic opportunistic infection (occurs in 28% of patients with AIDS). It usually presents as a focal cerebral abscess.
- Cryptococcal meningitis—*Cryptococcus neoformans* is the third most common infectious

205

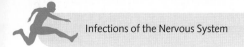

agent causing neurologic disease in AIDS. Classical clinical markers of meningitis may be absent. Pyrexia and headache, or even purely nonspecific symptoms, may be the only sign.

- Progressive multifocal leucoencephalopathy (PML)—caused by JC papovavirus, resulting in central demyelination which is relentlessly progressive and with a dismal prognosis.
- Cytomegalovirus (CMV)—can cause a retinitis, myelitis, and encephalitis.
- Herpes simplex type II—myelitis.
- Varicella-zoster—radiculitis and encephalitis.
- Other infections—*Candida*, *Aspergillus*, and *coccidioides* may affect the CNS.

Neoplasia
HIV infection may cause:
- Primary CNS lymphoma—presents as other mass lesions (occurs in 1.5% of AIDS patients as compared with 0.2% of other immunocompromised patients).
- Other malignancies—e.g., spread from systemic non-Hodgkin's lymphoma or, rarely, metastases from Kaposi's sarcoma.

Peripheral nervous system involvement
Peripheral neuropathy
HIV may be associated with the following peripheral neuropathies:
- Distal symmetrical polyneuropathy—the most common type of neuropathy (10–30% of patients). It is usually a late feature, with pain and paresthesiae of the feet. Treatment is symptomatic.
- Chronic inflammatory demyelinating polyradiculoneuropathy (CIDP)—an early feature. It includes a subacute, predominantly motor polyneuropathy, affecting proximal muscles more than distal, without painful dysesthesia. Plasmapheresis may help unlike in forms of CIDP in non-HIV-positive patients.
- Guillain Barré syndrome (GBS)—the acute counterpart of CIDP. This is an early feature that can occur at seroconversion. It has the same clinical features as seronegative GBS but with a high CSF lymphocyte count. Plasmapheresis may help.
- Mononeuritis multiplex—nerve infarction leads to sudden-onset sensory and motor deficits. Herpes zoster radiculitis must be excluded.

Myopathy
Myopathies caused by HIV include:
- Polymyositis—indistinguishable from seronegative polymyositis. Immunosuppressive treatment results in improvement.
- Type-II-fiber muscle atrophy—frequent finding on biopsy in patients with proximal weakness and normal creatine kinase (CK), creatine phosphokinase (CPK) levels.

Poliomyelitis
Poliovirus is one of the enteroviruses and is a picornavirus (pico—small; rna—RNA).

The incidence of primary infection has been extremely low in the U.S. since immunization began in 1955, but many patients have residual disability following infection during the 1950s and before.

Poliomyelitis remains endemic in the tropics, occurring especially in late summer and autumn.

Mode of spread
Poliomyelitis is spread by the fecal–oral route and then enters the bloodstream, causing a viremia.

Neurologic involvement occurs in only some patients and targets the anterior horn cells of the spinal cord and the motor nuclei of the brainstem.

Clinical features
The incubation period is 10–14 days.

There is considerable variation in symptoms:
- Asymptomatic (95%)—with resultant immunity.
- Abortive poliomyelitis (4–5%)—a self-limiting illness with gastrointestinal and mild upper respiratory symptoms and pyrexia.
- Nonparalytic poliomyelitis (0.5%)—features of abortive poliomyelitis with meningism. Recovery is complete.
- Paralytic poliomyelitis (0.1%)—initially there are features of abortive poliomyelitis which subside and then recur with meningism and myalgia. There is subsequent asymmetrical paralysis with no sensory involvement. Respiratory failure is due to paralysis of the respiratory muscles. The lower limb or limbs are most commonly affected, especially in children. Bulbar symptoms can occur with cranial nerve involvement. When paralytic poliomyelitis occurs before puberty, the patient is often left with a wasted, shortened limb.

Diagnosis of paralytic poliomyelitis
Paralytic poliomyelitis is distinguished clinically from GBS and transverse myelitis by the lack of sensory signs and the asymmetry.

CSF findings are similar to those in other viral meningitides (raised protein, increased number of lymphocytes, and normal glucose), but there are usually increased numbers of neutrophils initially.

The virus may be grown from throat swabs, stool, and CSF, and paired serology will show a rising titer.

Treatment of paralytic poliomyelitis
Patients with paralytic poliomyelitis should be isolated and contacts immunized. Other measures include:
- Careful nursing, as for all paralyzed patients, to prevent bed sores.
- Physiotherapy to avoid deformities.
- Fluid and electrolyte replacement.

Respiratory failure requires artificial ventilation.

Prognosis
Lack of ventilatory support for respiratory paralysis is the usual cause of death, but otherwise mortality rates are very low. Improvement in muscle power can commence a week after paralysis and continue for up to a year. Bulbar palsies recover the best. Some muscles may remain permanently paralyzed and fasciculations may persist.

In affected limbs in children, bone growth is retarded, resulting in a wasted, shortened limb.

Vaccination
Routine immunization from 2 months of age occurs in North America.

Up to 1963, Salk (inactivated) vaccine was used. Since then, the Sabin (live, attenuated) vaccine has been used. It is given orally in three doses, one month apart, starting at the age of 2 months, and then a reinforcing dose is given at school-entry age.

Note: Live virus will be excreted in the stool after immunization; therefore, great care must be taken to avoid transmission of infection to immunocompromised and nonvaccinated individuals.

Postpolio syndrome
A deterioration in function with atrophy in the affected as well as unaffected limbs can occur many years after the primary infection (usually between 20 and 40 years).

The cause is uncertain, but it may represent the normal aging process (i.e., loss of anterior horn cells)

with the symptoms accentuated by the prior reduction in anterior horn cell number caused by the original infection.

Lyme disease
The causative agent in Lyme disease is the spirochete *Borrelia burgdorferi*, which is transmitted by the tick *Ixodes dammini*.

The organism is prevalent throughout North America (e.g., Lyme, Connecticut, where the disease was first recognized) and Europe.

Clinical features
The clinical course of Lyme disease can be divided into three stages.

Stage 1 begins 3–30 days after the tick bite and consists of a relapsing remitting pyrexia and arthralgia, with a characteristic bull's-eye skin lesion (erythema migrans) developing at the site of the bite. This stage resolves after about 4 weeks.

Stage 2 occurs a few weeks or months after stage 1 and consists of neurologic (15%) or cardiac symptoms (10%), which can last up to 8 weeks. Neurologic manifestations include:
- Subacute lymphocytic meningitis—often mild and self-limiting but can recur if not treated.
- Subacute encephalitis—often mild and self-limiting.
- Cranial nerve involvement.
- Peripheral neuropathy with painful radiculitis.

Stage 3 occurs several months or years later and consists of recurrent and often erosive arthritis. Signs of diffuse CNS involvement may also develop, with focal encephalitis, seizures, behavioral disorders, and a multiple-sclerosis-like illness.

Diagnosis
Clinical features and epidemiologic considerations are indicative. Serologic techniques are highly effective. Cultures often give a low yield.

Treatment
Treatment consists of the following:
- Stage 1: oral antibiotics (doxycycline or amoxicillin).
- Stages 2 and 3: high-dose intravenous penicillin or ceftriaxone for 14 days. This shortens the course of neurologic illness and prevents further parenchymal damage.

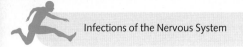

Prognosis

Focal deficits that do not improve after treatment and normalization of the CSF indicate fixed parenchymal damage and are hence unlikely ever to improve.

Creutzfeldt–Jakob disease (CJD)

CJD is an extremely rare disease that has received public awareness recently because of the possibility that the equivalent disease in cattle—bovine spongiform encephalitis (BSE)—may be transmissible to humans.

Transmission

CJD, BSE, and similar diseases (scrapie in sheep and kuru, which is found in Papua New Guinea) are transmitted by a protein (the prion protein) that is found within the nervous and, to a lesser extent, lymphatic systems of affected humans or animals.

The transformed, pathogenic prion protein is resistant to formalin, heat, irradiation, and procedures that modify nucleic acids.

CJD is not contagious but is infectious. It can be transmitted experimentally, and there are a number of examples of iatrogenic transfer (e.g., human pituitary-derived growth hormone given to growth-retarded children and transfer via corneal grafts).

There is no evidence of transmission via blood products or whole organ transplantation or across the placenta.

Incidence

In the U.S., there are 200 new cases per year. CJD affects 1 person per million worldwide.

However, since 1994, there have been reports a new atypical variant of CJD in the U.K., all of which have occurred in persons under the age of 42 years (mean age 27 years), and this has spurred the government's involvement and public concern.

Features of classic CJD

Classic CJD has a long incubation period, up to several years, and usually presents in the sixth decade of life.

It is characterized by the triad of:

- Dementia—rapid onset and progressive, with ultimate loss of language function.
- Myoclonus—brief, shock-like involuntary movements, often exaggerated on being startled.

- A characteristic but nonspecific EEG abnormality—generalized slowing or pseudoperiodic sharp waves.

The disease is rapidly progressive and invariably fatal, often within 6 months from the onset of symptoms. Brain pathology shows characteristic spongiform (vacuolated) changes in the brain.

Features of new variant CJD

New variant CJD is a young-onset form which was not seen until 1994.

Clinical features include behavioral change, ataxia, cognitive impairment, and a tendency to a more prolonged duration of illness (up to 23 months).

The EEG is not typical of classic sporadic CJD. Brain pathology shows marked spongiform change and extensive amyloid plaques.

Diagnosis

Diagnosis is based on:
- Clinical picture and EEG.
- Spinal fluid—14–3-3 protein is suggestive, but there are false positives and false negatives.
- Brain biopsy and tonsil biopsy in new variant CJD.
- Autopsy—unfortunately, the definitive diagnosis is often made this way.

Newer techniques to detect the prion protein are increasingly being used.

Treatment

There is no treatment for CJD. Sedative or antipsychotics can help control behavior. Patients should be encouraged to make a living will or advance directives.

Comment

The current opinion from the Spongiform Encephalopathy Advisory Committee (SEAC), concerning the young cases of new variant CJD, is that "in the absence of any credible alternative, the most likely explanation at present is that these cases are linked to exposure to BSE before the Specified Bovine Offal (SBO) ban was introduced in 1989." The SBO ban prohibits the use of the tissues most likely to contain the infective agent of BSE in products for human consumption. These tissues include brain, spinal cord, thymus, tonsils, spleen, intestines, and, more recently, bones.

34. Multiple Sclerosis

Multiple sclerosis (MS) is a common disease in North America and Europe. There are multiple areas of demyelination within the central nervous system (CNS). The episodes of demyelination are separated in time and place, and classically the disease runs a relapsing-remitting course.

Incidence

MS occurs worldwide but is far more common in temperate climates, with the incidence increasing proportionally with the distance from the equator. This applies in the northern and southern hemispheres. In the U.S., MS occurs more frequently above the 37th parallel, which runs from Newport News, Virginia, to Santa Cruz, California, including the northern border of North Carolina and the northern border of Arizona. Above this line, the prevalence is 110–140 cases/100,000; below the line, the prevalence is 47–78 cases/100,000.

Interestingly, on moving from a high-prevalence area to a low-prevalence area prior to puberty, the risk of developing the disease takes on the rate of the low-prevalence area; however, if such a move is made following puberty, the risk of the high-prevalence area is retained.

The disease usually occurs in young adults, the peak age of onset being between 20 and 30 years. More females than males are affected.

Pathogenesis

A large number of theories exist regarding the pathogenesis of MS, since the exact cause is uncertain. Immunologic mechanisms undoubtedly play a role, although the causation is probably multifactorial.

Immunologic mechanisms
Evidence points toward the presence of immunoregulatory defects in MS. Recent research has suggested that cytokines may play a critical role

in the pathophysiology, both by regulating aberrant autoimmune responses and by mediating myelin damage.

Familial factors
There is an increased familial incidence of MS, with a relative of an affected individual having a 20-fold increased risk of developing the disease. There is not a clearcut pattern of inheritance but there is a positive association with HLA-A3, B7, B18, DR2, and DW2.

Infection
Because of the presence of a defective immunologic response in patients with MS, a viral etiology in a susceptible host has been suggested. Raised titers to many common viruses have been found in the serum and cerebrospinal fluid (CSF) of MS patients, but attempts to induce MS experimentally with viruses have been unsuccessful.

Biochemical mechanisms
No biochemical effect has been demonstrated. Myelin is normal prior to breakdown. Reports that excessive dietary fats or fat malabsorption are important have not been substantiated.

Pathology

Areas of demyelination are found in the white matter of the brain and spinal cord. These areas are called plaques. The lesions lie in close relationship to postcapillary venules (perivenular).

There is a particular predilection for the:
- Periventricular region of the brain.
- Brainstem and its cerebellar connections (including medial longitudinal fasciculus).
- Cervical cord.
- Optic nerves.

There is myelin destruction with relative preservation of axons. An inflammatory infiltrate containing mononuclear cells and lymphocytes is

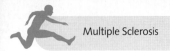
found. Interstitial edema occurs in acute lesions. Remyelination is rare and the mechanism of functional recovery is uncertain.

Clinical features

MS can present in a multitude of ways, and no single presentation is diagnostic. For instance, a young woman with a history of two or more episodes of CNS dysfunction that have remitted would be highly suggestive.

Three main patterns of disease progression are recognized:

- Relapsing and remitting—symptom exacerbations followed by improvements.
- Secondary progressive—the disease starts with a relapsing–remitting picture, but recovery from each successive relapse becomes less and less complete, causing residual disability.
- Primary progressive—little or no recovery from relapses, with cumulative disability.

There is a marked variability in the disease progress, but by 15 years, 30% of patients are still working and 40% are still walking.

The most common presentations are discussed below.

Optic and retrobulbar neuritis

Optic neuritis presents as subacute visual loss, usually unilateral, associated with a central scotoma and pain on ocular movement. Recovery is usual over a few weeks. The ophthalmological findings depend on whether the lesion is in the optic nerve head (optic neuritis; papillitis) or in the optic nerve behind the eye (retrobulbar neuritis). In the former, a pink swollen disc is seen, whereas in the latter, the disc looks normal.

Papillitis can look similar to papilledema through an ophthalmoscope. Papillitis causes early and profound loss in vision, with a central scotoma. In papilledema, visual deterioration is a late feature and there is an enlargement of the blind spot.

There are usually no residual symptoms following optic neuritis, although a relative afferent pupillary defect (Fig. 34.1), small scotomata, and defects in color vision may be demonstrated. Following an attack, optic atrophy (pale disc) often develops.

Optic neuritis may be an isolated event, it may occur simultaneously with a transverse myelitis (Devic's syndrome), or it may be a forerunner for further episodes of CNS demyelination (i.e., MS). Up to 70% of cases fall into the last category.

In some patients, optic nerve demyelination may be asymptomatic and only be discovered clinically by the presence of optic atrophy or by the use of visual evoked potentials (see p. 211 and Chapter 19).

Brainstem presentation

There is a predilection in MS for demyelination to affect the cerebellar connections and the medial longitudinal fasciculus (see Fig. 24.3) in the brainstem.

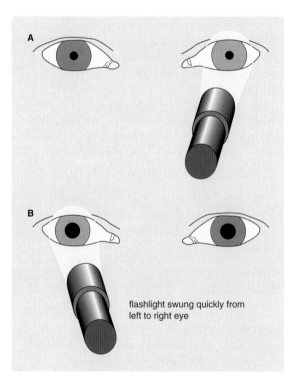

Fig. 34.1 Afferent pupillary defect in right eye: light shone into the normal left eye (A) causes consensual constriction of both pupils, but both pupils consensually dilate somewhat when the torch swings to the abnormal right eye (B). Less light gets into the afferent arc of the reflex, due to the right optic nerve lesion.

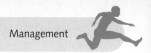

Classic presentations include:

- Diplopia—often due to internuclear ophthalmoplegia (failure of adduction of one eye, with coarse nystagmus of the other abducting eye on lateral gaze), caused by a lesion of the medial longitudinal fasciculus. This may be unilateral or, more commonly, bilateral.
- Nystagmus (due to cerebellar disease).
- Vertigo.
- Dysarthria—often cerebellar.
- Numbness or paresthesias.
- Dysphagia.
- Ataxia.
- Pyramidal signs—with involvement of the corticospinal tracts.

Spinal cord lesion (myelopathy)

A spinal cord lesion is a common presentation and results in a spastic paraparesis or tetraparesis, often with tonic spasms of the limbs. There is associated difficulty walking and sensory loss. Bladder symptoms are common.

Lhermitte's sign, in which there is a brief, electric-shock-like sensation down the limbs on flexion of the neck, may be present.

The symptoms and signs of MS tend to get worse with heat (e.g., in the bath or during hot weather) (Uhthoff's phenomenon).

Differential diagnosis

Initial presentation may cause diagnostic difficulty, but few other conditions follow a similar subsequent pattern of relapsing and remitting CNS disease. The exceptions are Behçet's disease, CNS sarcoidosis, and systemic lupus erythematosus (SLE).

There are multiple causes of optic neuritis, brainstem syndromes, and myelopathy, and these must be excluded on initial presentation.

Investigations

There is no diagnostic test for MS, but the clinical suspicion is supported by the following three tests.

Magnetic resonance imaging (MRI)

Computed tomography (CT) scans do not accurately pick up areas of demyelination, whereas MRI is far more sensitive at showing this white-matter disease. Hyperintense lesions are seen on T2-weighted images.

Widespread abnormalities are often seen at presentation, despite the disease clinically appearing as unifocal and new-onset.

Similar hyperintense lesions may be seen in vascular and granulomatous disorders.

Cerebrospinal fluid (CSF) examination

A mild lymphocyte pleocytosis may be present, especially during relapses. The protein may be slightly elevated. However, the presence of oligoclonal bands in the CSF but not in the serum is highly suggestive of MS.

Oligoclonal bands may also be found in many chronic infective or inflammatory conditions involving the CNS.

Evoked potentials
Visual evoked potentials (VEPs)

If there has been demyelination at any time along the optic nerve (i.e., optic neuritis), whether symptomatic or asymptomatic, the conduction of visual images (usually a changing checkerboard) to the occipital cortex will be delayed. The normal response takes about 100 milliseconds.

Somatosensory evoked potentials (SSEPs)

Measurement of SSEPs may detect a delay in central sensory pathways.

Brainstem auditory evoked potentials (BAEPs)

Measurement of BAEPs during auditory testing, may detect brainstem lesions.

Management

Treatments for the disease process
Anti-inflammatory treatment

Steroidal therapy, usually given intravenously as methylprednisolone (high dose for 3 days), is the mainstay treatment used for relapses. This may shorten the duration of the relapse but does not appear to affect outcome.

Suppression or modulation of the immune system

Interferon-β 1a (Avonex, Rebif) and 1b (Betaseron) are currently being used, but with mixed results.

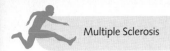

Glateramer acetate (Capoxone), an amino acid mixture that modifies the immune system, reduces exacerbations and disability. The relapse rate is modestly reduced, but it is not yet clear whether these agents significantly slow the progression of disability. These agents are given by injection.

Symptomatic treatment
Spasticity
Spasticity can be a considerable problem, especially if painful spasms develop. Drugs such as baclofen, dantrolene, diazepam, and tizanidine can be helpful. Care must be taken not to reduce the tone too much, as some patients require the increased tone to walk.

Contractures may be prevented with physiotherapy.

Bladder dysfunction
Anticholinergic drugs may help incontinence. Intermittent self-cathetherization or a permanent urinary catheter may be required. Intravesical capsaicin has also been shown to help.

Prevention and early treatment of urinary tract infections are important because the symptoms and signs can deteriorate with intercurrent infection.

Paroxysmal symptoms
Some patients develop tonic muscle spasms, burning dysesthetic pains, and other brief brainstem syndromes that may be helped by carbamazepine, phenytoin, or gabapentin, acting as membrane stabilizers.

Intention tremor
The cerebellar tremor can be quite disabling and can sometimes be reduced with clonazepam.

Fatigue
Amantadine (Symmetrel) or modafinil (Provigil) may be used when adequate diet and daily exercise do not help.

Other central demyelinating diseases

A number of other rarer diseases can cause demyelination within the CNS, but their presentation is very different from MS. These include:
- Acute demyelinating encephalomyelitis (ADEM).
- Progressive multifocal leukoencephalopathy (PML).
- Leukodystrophies—metachromatic leukodystrophy, adrenoleukodystrophy.

35. Systemic Disease and the Nervous System

Neurologic complications of endocrine disease

Diabetes mellitus

Diabetes mellitus is by far the most common endocrinologic and metabolic cause of neurologic symptoms and signs involving the whole nervous system.

Coma

Coma can result during hypoglycemia, or during ketotic or nonketotic hyperglycemia. All patients in a coma should immediately have their glucose measured.

Cerebrovascular disease

Patients with diabetes have a higher risk of developing a wide range of cerebrovascular disease than does the general population. This includes large-vessel (e.g., middle cerebral artery occlusion) and small-vessel diseases (e.g., pseudobulbar palsy syndrome and multi-infarct dementia).

Visual loss

Visual loss in diabetes may be due to retinal disease and hemorrhage, cataracts, or vascular disease.

Peripheral nerve lesions

Peripheral neuropathy is a very common finding in diabetes. Different types exist. The most common are:
- Distal symmetrical polyneuropathy.
- Proximal motor neuropathy (diabetic amyotrophy).
- Compression neuropathies (e.g., carpal tunnel syndrome).
- Multifocal neuropathy (mononeuritis multiplex)—diabetes is the most common cause of this syndrome, which may may affect peripheral nerves in the limbs or certain cranial nerves, especially the third, sixth, and seventh (see Chapter 24).
- Autonomic neuropathy.

Thyrotoxicosis

Clinical features of Graves' disease often include exophthalmos with ophthalmoplegia. This is due to infiltration of the periorbital muscles.

A high-frequency tremor is characteristic and a proximal myopathy may be present. The severe weight loss, with muscle atrophy and brisk reflexes that may be present in severe cases, can be difficult to differentiate from motor neuron disease. This resolves rapidly with treatment of the hyperthyroidism.

In addition, atrial fibrillation is common and may result in embolic cerebral infarction.

Hypothyroidism

Carpal tunnel syndrome is common in hypothyroidism. Myopathy, neuropathy, and "myxedema madness" are extremely rare.

Cushing's disease and syndrome

Whether corticosteroid excess is due to a pituitary tumor, adrenal production, or exogenous steroid therapy, similar neurologic features may result. These include proximal myopathy and psychosis.

A pituitary tumour may cause optic chiasmal compression with a resultant bitemporal hemianopia.

Addison's disease

Addison's disease causes mental and physical lethargy. A mild proximal myopathy may be present.

Acromegaly

Initially, in acromegaly, there may be an increase in muscle strength, but a proximal myopathy follows. Optic chiasmal compression causes bitemporal hemianopia. Carpal tunnel syndrome and peroneal nerve entrapment are common. Diabetes mellitus often develops and thus all its neurologic sequelae may be seen.

Neurologic complications of renal disease

Encephalopathy
Encephalopathy occurs secondary to uremia. If the development of uremia is slow, this results in poor concentration and memory impairment. Misperceptions and visual hallucinations are common. Rapid development of uremia can cause a severe encephalopathy, with deterioration of conscious level, coma, seizures, and focal signs.

Electroencephalography may show a generalized encephalopathic picture, epileptic activity, or triphasic waves (also common in hepatic encephalopathy).

Movement disorders associated with renal failure
Movement disorders associated with renal failure include:
- Myoclonus or limb tremor.
- Asterixis—a nonspecific phenomenon in which there is a coarse flapping tremor when the hands are outstretched and the wrists hyperextended. It also occurs with hypercapnia and liver failure.

Other central nervous system signs associated with renal failure
Other signs associated with renal failure include:
- Transient focal signs—a reversible hemiparesis can occur with dialysis. It can alternate sides and appears to be a metabolic phenomenon rather than ischemic, as it progresses over a few hours.
- Stiffness and rigidity—usually involving axial muscles, with a board-like neck.
- Gait disturbance—usually part of a slowly developing encephalopathy, with marked unsteadiness.
- Seizures—there is a high incidence of seizures associated with renal failure.

Peripheral nervous system involvement in renal failure
Peripheral axonal neuropathy
Peripheral axonal neuropathy begins with burning and tingling pains in the feet, and restless legs. As it progresses, there is the development of a symmetrical sensorimotor neuropathy with absent ankle jerks.

The neuropathy is usually mainly sensory, and profound weakness may be due to another cause (e.g., hyperkalemia).

There may be reversal or lack of progression of the neuropathy with stabilization of the disease or with transplantation.

Other complications of chronic renal failure
Other complications of chronic renal failure include confusional states and dementia in patients on dialysis, secondary amyloidosis, and side effects of immunosuppression in renal transplant cases. A range of infections may occur, particularly fungal, and lymphoma of the central nervous system develops in 5% of transplant case. Cyclosporin can cause seizures, encephalopathy, neuropathy, and myopathy.

Neurologic complications of connective tissue disease

There are a wide variety of conditions that cause inflammatory changes in connective tissue, especially of blood vessels. Many of the features overlap. The neurologic complications often relate to the vascular changes.

Systemic lupus erythematosus (SLE)
The multisystem disorder SLE may be complicated by seizures, psychosis, cerebrovascular disease (large and small vessel), movement disorders, extraocular muscle palsies, multifocal neuropathy multiplex (mononeuritis multiplex), and polymyositis.

A central demyelinating variant that mimics multiple sclerosis may occur.

Rheumatoid arthritis
Rheumatoid arthritis is associated with carpal tunnel syndrome, multifocal neuropathy, muscle atrophy, and the serious complication of high cervical spinal cord compression. Cerebral arteritis is very rare.

Treatment with penicillamine causes a myasthenic syndrome in some patients. Prolonged steroid use may cause a proximal myopathy.

Polyarteritis nodosa

Polyarteritis nodosa causes a panarteritis with local thrombosis and occasionally rupture with microhemorrhages.

The most common neurologic manifestations are due to peripheral nerve infarction, causing multifocal neuropathy. Cranial nerve palsies and cerebrovascular disease are less common.

Polymyositis

This inflammatory muscle disease has been discussed in Chapter 30. It is associated with connective tissue disease in up to 25% of cases.

Sjögren's syndrome

A wide variety of neurologic manifestations can occur with Sjögren's syndrome, including peripheral neuropathy, entrapment syndromes, myelopathy, proximal myopathy, and meningoencephalitis. In addition, an isolated trigeminal neuropathy can occur.

Neurologic complications of neoplastic disease

Neurologic manifestations of neoplasia (apart from primary nervous system tumors) can arise from cerebral metastases, nonmetastatic causes (often antibody-mediated), or be due to the side effects of radiotherapy or the drugs used in chemotherapy.

Here, discussion will be limited to conditions arising from nonmetastatic causes. In these conditions, there is no evidence of metastases or infiltration by the tumor. They include:

- Peripheral neuropathy—a common finding in a variety of tumors, especially those of the bronchus and kidney. It is usually sensory, but a motor neuropathy can also occur.
- Limbic encephalitis—occurs in small-cell carcinoma of the lung and is associated with anti-Hu antibodies.
- Cerebellar syndrome—occurs in ovarian tumors and is associated with anti-Purkinje-cell antibodies (anti-Yo).
- Dermatomyositis—is associated with underlying carcinoma in up to 10% of cases (see Chapter 30).
- Lambert–Eaton myasthenic syndrome—occurs with small-cell carcinoma of the bronchus and is associated with antibodies directed against presynaptic voltage-gated calcium channels (see Chapter 29).

Neurologic complications associated with cardiac disease

Atrial fibrillation is the most common cardiac risk factor for stroke, especially when there is associated heart failure or left atrial enlargement.

During or following myocardial infarction, cerebral hypoperfusion may occur. There may be subsequent embolism from mural thrombus. The routine use of thrombolytic agents reduces the risk of the latter but increases the risk of cerebral hemorrhage.

Disease of the mitral and aortic valves increases the risk of cerebral emboli, especially with infective endocarditis.

Congenital heart disease is also associated with neurologic disease. There is a high incidence of cerebral aneurysms with coarctation of the aorta. Cyanotic heart diseases can cause chronic cerebral anoxia.

Abrupt changes in cardiac rhythm, usually profound bradycardia, present as sudden faintness or loss of consciousness (Stokes–Adams attacks). These are typically brief, with more rapid recovery than from seizure. Ventricular tachycardias are a less common cause.

215

36. Effects of Deficiency Diseases and Toxins on the Nervous System

Deficiency diseases

Nutritional deficiencies are particularly common in developing countries but do occur in developed countries due to food fads, alcoholism, and malabsorption syndromes. The most common conditions will be described below.

Vitamin B$_1$ (thiamine) deficiency

Deficiency of vitamin B$_1$ causes beriberi or Wernicke–Korsakoff syndrome.

Beriberi

Beriberi is caused by a staple diet of polished rice and results in either a polyneuropathy (dry beriberi) or marked generalized edema with ascites and pleural effusions (wet beriberi).

Wernicke–Korsakoff syndrome

Wernicke–Korsakoff syndrome is more common in the Western world than beriberi and is caused primarily by chronic alcoholism with poor dietary intake of thiamine.

The syndrome is composed of an acute phase (Wernicke's encephalopathy) and a chronic phase (Korsakoff's psychosis).

The typical triad of Wernicke's encephalopathy includes:

- Ocular signs—with nystagmus and ophthalmoplegia.
- Ataxia—with a broad-based gait, and cerebellar signs in the limbs, especially the legs.
- Confusion—with disorientation, apathy, agitation, amnesia, stupor, and coma.

In chronic cases, a slower amnesic syndrome develops, with selective impairment of short-term memory, which is compensated for by confabulation (Korsakoff's psychosis).

The pathology of Wernicke–Korsakoff syndrome involves symmetrical damage to the mamillary bodies, thalamus, and periaqueductal gray matter.

Treatment for Wernicke's encephalopathy is intravenous thiamine followed by a normal diet and continued oral thiamine. Korsakoff's psychosis is treated with oral thiamine and a normal diet.

In thiamine deficiency, glucose is inadequately metabolized and lactate and pyruvate accumulate. It is therefore essential to give thiamine immediately to any patient with suspected thiamine deficiency, before giving any sugar-containing substance, especially 5% dextrose or dextrose saline.

Vitamin B$_6$ (pyridoxine) deficiency

Vitamin B$_6$ deficiency causes a mainly sensory neuropathy and may be precipitated during isoniazid therapy for tuberculosis. Pyridoxine supplements should therefore be given when isoniazid is prescribed.

Vitamin B$_{12}$ deficiency

Deficiency of vitamin B$_{12}$ may, rarely, result from nutritional deficiency (e.g., vegans) but is more often caused by malabsorption. The usual causes are pernicious anemia, gastrectomy, and diseases of the terminal ileum (e.g., Crohn's disease, blind-loop syndrome). Up to 25% of patients with neurologic damage caused by vitamin B$_{12}$ deficiency do not have hematologic abnormalities (i.e., macrocytic megaloblastic anemia).

The condition includes damage to the peripheral nerves, dorsal columns, and corticospinal tracts bilaterally and is called subacute combined degeneration of the cord.

Treatment with intramuscular vitamin B$_{12}$ must be started promptly. If treatment is initiated early,

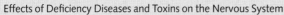

Toxins and their neurologic effects		
Toxin	**Clinical effect**	
	Acute	**Chronic**
arsenic	encephalopathy	peripheral neuropathy
lead	encephalopathy (especially in children)	encephalopathy and peripheral neuropathy (especially motor)
manganese	encephalopathy	parkinsonism
mercury	headache, tremor	ataxia, peripheral neuropathy, encephalopathy, psychosis
tin	amnesia, seizures	encephalomyelopathy
toluene	narcosis	ataxia, encephalopathy
perchloroethylene	narcosis	peripheral neuropathy, encephalopathy
organophosphates	cholinergic crisis	ataxia, paralysis, peripheral neuropathy

Fig. 36.1 Toxins and their neurologic effects.

there can be complete recovery; if delayed, the progression may be halted but there is little reversal. The condition can be made dramatically worse by giving folic acid without vitamin B_{12}.

Folic acid deficiency

It has been suggested that deficiency of folic acid (folate) causes neuropathy and dementia. However, the evidence is somewhat conflicting, and folate deficiency is often found on a background of either chronic alcohol abuse with poor nutritional intake or malabsorption syndromes, when neurologic conditions may be arising from other causes.

Nicotinic acid deficiency

Nicotinic acid deficiency causes pellagra and is found in areas where the staple diet is maize. The clinical features include dermatitis, diarrhea, and dementia.

Vitamin E deficiency

Vitamin E is a fat-soluble vitamin that can become deficient with malabsorption syndromes, especially in cystic fibrosis, celiac disease, and diseases in which there is a reduced bile-salt pool. There is a rare familial fat-malabsorption syndrome with abetalipoproteinemia.

Vitamin E deficiency causes primarily an ataxic syndrome, with areflexia and loss of vibration sense and proprioception, but sparing of cutaneous sensation.

Treatment is with oral vitamin E.

Toxins

There are numerous toxins capable of causing neurologic symptoms. The most common are listed in Fig. 36.1.

37. Hereditary Conditions of the Nervous System

Neurocutaneous syndromes

A number of inherited conditions involve disorders of organs derived from the ectoderm, causing tumors (benign and malignant), hamartomas, and lesions in the skin and nervous system. Only the most common are outlined below.

Neurofibromatosis

There are a number of different types of neurofibromatosis, but types 1 (peripheral predominance) and 2 (central predominance) are the most important.

Neurofibromatosis type 1 (von Recklinghausen's disease)

Neurofibromatosis type 1 is an autosomal dominant condition caused by a defect on chromosome 17, with an incidence of 1 in 4,000.

Clinically, it is characterized by (Fig. 37.1):
- Neurofibromas—lying along peripheral nerves.
- Café-au-lait spots—multiple pale-brown macules, especially on the trunk. They are found in the normal population, but more than five in an individual is abnormal.
- Cutaneous fibromas (molluscum fibrosum)—subcutaneous, soft, often pedunculated, pink tumors, usually multiple.
- Axillary freckling.
- Lisch nodules—small hamartomas of the iris.

Other associated features include:
- Neural tumors—there is a higher incidence of neural tumors than in the general population (e.g., meningioma, acoustic schwannoma, glioma, spinal root neurofibroma).
- Skeletal abnormalities—50% of patients have a scoliosis. There may be bone hypertrophy underlying subperiosteal neurofibromas.
- Endocrine abnormalities—associated pheochromocytoma, medullary carcinoma of the thyroid, multiple endocrine neoplasia.

- Local gigantism of a limb ("elephant man").
- Mental retardation and epilepsy—occurs in 10–15% of patients.
- Renal artery stenosis.
- Obstructive cardiomyopathy.
- Pulmonary fibrosis.

Neurofibromatosis type 2

Neurofibromatosis type 2 is an autosomal dominant condition caused by a defect on chromosome 22, with an incidence of 1 in 50,000.

Clinically, it is characterized by few skin and skeletal manifestations and the presence of bilateral eighth nerve schwannomas (acoustic neuromas). Other intracranial and intraspinal tumors are common.

Treatment

Intracranial tumours require excision and, if necessary, radiotherapy. Cosmetic surgery may be required for the cutaneous manifestations. Genetic counseling is important.

Tuberous sclerosis

Tuberous sclerosis is an autosomal dominant condition with an incidence of 1 in 30,000.

It is characterized by skin lesions, especially adenoma sebaceum on the face (Fig. 37.2), epilepsy, and varying degrees of mental retardation.

In addition to the nodular lesions on the cheeks (adenoma sebaceum), skin manifestations include depigmented patches (ash-leaf spot), "shagreen" patches, and subungual fibromas. Slowly expanding cerebral tumors may occur (hamartomatous "tubers" and astrocytomas). Systemic tumors may affect the kidney, lung, or muscle.

Treatment

The epilepsy is often quite resistant to treatment. Surgery may be required for large cerebral tumors, especially if hydrocephalus is developing. Careful regular evaluation of these patients must be made to catch the development of any of the complications of the disease.

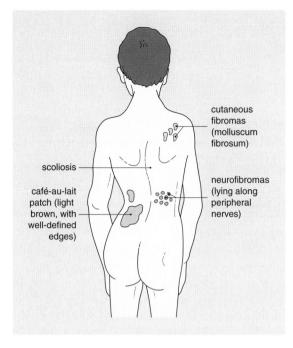

Fig. 37.1 Cutaneous manifestations of neurofibromatosis type 1.

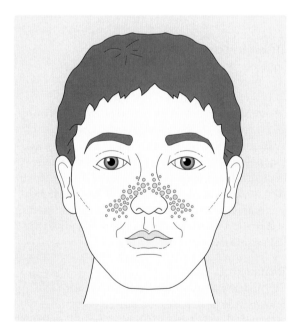

Fig. 37.2 Adenoma sebaceum—classic raised reddish nodules found over the nose and cheeks in tuberous sclerosis.

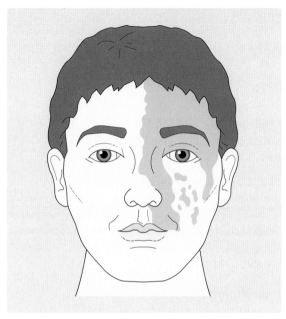

Fig. 37.3 Port-wine nevus in Sturge–Weber syndrome.

Sturge–Weber syndrome

Sturge–Weber syndrome has no clear inheritance pattern. It is characterized by an extensive port-wine nevus on one side of the face (Fig. 37.3), usually within the first and second divisions of the trigeminal nerve, and an underlying leptomeningeal angioma. There may be atrophy of the affected hemisphere, epilepsy, and congenital glaucoma.

If epilepsy is sufficiently intractable, lobectomy or even hemispherectomy may be required. The early removal of the surface lesion remains controversial.

Spinocerebellar degeneration

A large number of inherited conditions produce varying clinical pictures of spinocerebellar degeneration. Two of the more common conditions are outlined below.

Friedreich's ataxia

Friedreich's ataxia is an autosomal recessive condition caused by a trinucleotide repeat on chromosome 9. The phenotype depends on the number of trinucleotide repeats. The abnormal protein is called frataxin and is found in the spinal cord, heart, and pancreas. Little of the protein is found in the cerebellum or cerebrum.

Within the spinal cord there is progressive degeneration of the posterior columns, corticospinal tracts, and dorsal and ventral spinocerebellar tracts. Difficulty in walking begins around the age of 12 years. Death is usual before the age of 40, often from cardiac complications.

Clinical features include:
- Ataxia—starting in the legs, spreading to the arms. Dysarthria is delayed for at least 5 years.
- Neuropathy—absent ankle jerks.
- Absent joint-position sense and vibration.
- Pyramidal signs—upgoing plantar responses (despite absent ankle jerks).
- Skeletal abnormalities—pes cavus and scoliosis.
- Cardiomyopathy and arrhythymias.
- Optic atrophy—occurs in 30% of patients.

Ataxia telangiectasia
Ataxia telangiectasia is an autosomal recessive disorder causing progressive cerebellar ataxia, ocular and cutaneous telangiectasia, and immunodeficiency. Death is usual by the third decade, from infection or lymphoreticular malignancy.

Inherited neuropathies
See Chapter 28.

Inborn errors of metabolism

Numerous rare metabolic conditions can cause nervous system abnormalities. Two of these will be discussed briefly; others are listed in Figs 37.4 and 37.5.

Porphyria
The porphyrias comprise a heterogeneous group of disorders of heme synthesis, causing overproduction of porphyrins.

Acute intermittent porphyria, an autosomal dominant disorder occurring in adult life, can cause neurologic complications. It can be precipitated by certain drugs or alcohol.

Clinical features and their frequency are as follows:
- Abdominal pain—90%.
- Peripheral neuropathy—70%; usually an acute motor neuropathy that can present like Guillain Barré syndrome.
- Hypertension and tachycardia—70%.
- Psychiatric disturbance—50%.

Diagnosis can be made by screening for urine for porphobilinogen levels. However, testing the blood

Metabolic encephalomyopathies
Disorders of phenylalanine
phenylketonuria
Disorders of sulfur amino acid metabolism
homocystinuria
Disorders of branched-chain amino acids
maple syrup urine disease
Organic acidemias
carnitine deficiency
methylmalonic acid deficiency
carnitine palmityl transferase deficiency
acyl CoA dehydrogenase deficiency
Lactic acidosis
pyruvate dehydrogenase deficiency
Leigh's disease
Disorders of sugar metabolism
galactosemia
Disorders of purine metabolism
Lesch-Nyhan syndrome
xanthine oxidase deficiency
Disorders of pyrimidine metabolism
xeroderma pigmentosum
Porphyrias
Lipoprotein deficiencies
abetalipoproteinemia
Tangier disease
Disorders of copper metabolism
Wilson's disease
Menke's kinky-hair syndrome
Mitochondrial encephalomyopathies
MELAS/MERRF/CPEO
Peroxisomal disorders
infantile Refsum's disease
adrenoleukodystrophy

Fig. 37.4 Some examples of metabolic encephalomyopathies. (CPEO, chronic progressive external ophthalmoplegia; MELAS, myoclonic epilepsy and ragged red fibers; MERRF, mitochondrial encephalomyopathy, lactic acidosis, and stroke-like episodes.)

for reduced erythrocyte porphobilinogen deaminase and raised aminolevulinic acid synthetase is most sensitive.

Management is largely supportive, with a high carbohydrate intake, narcotics for pain, and hematin infusion. Any drugs that precipitate the condition should be avoided.

Wilson's disease (hepatolenticular degeneration)
Wilson's disease is a rare autosomal recessive disorder of copper metabolism. There is a deficiency of ceruloplasmin, which binds copper, resulting in

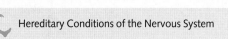

Metabolic storage diseases
Glycogen storage diseases
Pompe's disease
Cholesterol storage diseases
cerebrotendinous xanthomatosis
Neuronal ceroid lipofuscinosis
late onset (Kufs')
Mucopolysaccharidoses
Hurler's (type I)
Hunter's (type II)
Sphingolipidoses
gangliosidoses
GM1 gangliosidosis
GM2 gangliosidosis
Niemann–Pick disease
Gaucher's disease
Krabbe's disease
Fabry's disease
metachromatic leukodystrophy

Fig. 37.5 Metabolic storage diseases.

copper deposition in various organs, especially in the liver and the basal ganglia in the brain.

Clinical features include:

- Movement disorder—a wide range of movements can occur, including tremor, athetoid posturing, dystonic movements, and parkinsonism.
- Cirrhosis of the liver.
- Kayser–Fleischer ring—a fine brown deposition of copper in Descemet's membrane of the cornea, which may ultimately form a ring. This may be visible to the naked eye, but slit-lamp examination is usually necessary.

Diagnosis is by measurement of a low serum ceruloplasmin with elevated unbound copper. There is high urinary copper excretion, and liver biopsy may show massive copper deposition.

Treatment involves a lifelong low-copper diet and a chelating agent such as penicillamine. Liver transplantation is sometimes performed.

Index

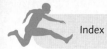

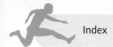

Index

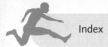

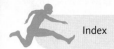

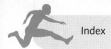

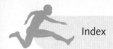

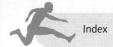

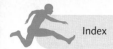

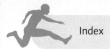

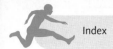

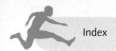